TOTAL RELAXATION

Healing Practices for
Body, Mind & Spirit

John R. Harvey, Ph.D.

KODANSHA INTERNATIONAL

NEW YORK • TOKYO • LONDON

This book is dedicated to my wife Dawn and my children, Nada, Jacob, Adam, and Sarah. Their love and support helped me to complete this book.

Kodansha America, Inc.
114 Fifth Avenue, New York, New York 10011, U.S.A.

Kodansha International Ltd.
17-14 Otowa 1-chome, Bunkyo-ku, Tokyo 112-8652, Japan

Published in 1998 by Kodansha America, Inc.

Library of Congress Cataloging-in-Publication Data
Harvey, John, 1945–
    Total relaxation / John R. Harvey.
        p. cm.
    ISBN 1-56836-224-2
    1. Relaxation. 2. Stress management. 3. Exercise therapy.
I. Title.
RA785.H375   1998
613.7'9—dc21   97-32360
                                                    CIP

Produced by becker&mayer!, Kirkland, Washington
www.beckermayer.com

Book design and illustration by Two Pollard Design
Art direction by Simon Sung
Edited by Jennifer Worick
Cover and interior images: Copyright © 1998 Photodisc Inc.

Book Manufactured in China
CD Mastered in Hong Kong

98 99 00 01 02   10 9 8 7 6 5 4 3 2 1

ACKNOWLEDGMENTS

I wish to acknowledge the inspiring work of those many contemporary physicians, psychologists, and healers who have developed and taught modern relaxation therapies. Acknowledgment must also go to those unknown teachers and healers who in the distant past developed relaxation techniques that have stood the test of time and are now available for all of us to use.

This book was inspired by the many patients who taught me that different relaxation techniques work for different people with different problems. Thanks also go to those students and seminar participants who told me that my information on relaxation needed to be available in a book. Thanks go to Swami Rama who inspired me with the statement, "Sit down and write and the words will come to you."

Thanks go to Deborah Baker, executive editor at Kodansha America, who guided me in shaping and editing this original manuscript into its present, more focused form. Thanks also go to Jennifer Worick of becker&mayer!, who skillfully and thoughtfully coordinated the production of this book.

I would also like to acknowledge the specific help of several colleagues. Dr. Phil Nuernberger of Mind Resources Technologies offered encouragement and advice throughout this project. Sue Logan, a wise and experienced physical therapist, provided technical and editorial comments for the chapters on muscular relaxation. Pastor Jon Buxton gave a very helpful review of the chapters on spiritual relaxation.

CONTENTS

chapter one

tension and

relaxation:

an introduction

"You just need to relax" must be the most frequently given words of advice. Doctors tell you to relax. Your spouse tells you to relax. Friends and coworkers tell you to relax. And late at night when you can't fall asleep because your muscles are wired tight and your mind is racing, you tell yourself you have to relax.

Yet to relax is easier said than done. Many questions arise. How do you relax? What techniques should you use? Should you exercise, join an aerobics class, swim, jog, meditate, visualize mountain scenery, or do breathing exercises? What really works? Which technique is right for you? When are you going to find time?

You might even have a subtle fear of relaxation; you may think that if you let go and relax, you won't get as much done. Relaxation might bring vulnerability. Or you may feel unable to relax.

This book is written to answer these questions, relieve these fears, and help you find relaxation techniques that work for you. Relaxation is a natural skill anyone can learn and use on a daily basis for great benefit. But before we learn relaxation techniques, let us explore the problem of tension and the benefits of relaxation.

THE PROBLEM OF TENSION

Some people notice tension in the back of the neck and

shoulders. Or a glance in the mirror reveals tension as a furrowed brow, a clenched jaw, or tight lips. Others experience tension internally as a nervous stomach, racing heart, shaky limbs, or sweaty palms. Or tension may be experienced in the mind as scattered, racing, and repetitive thoughts. Tension can be felt emotionally as fears, worries, and floating anxiety. It can occur on the spiritual level as a lack of purpose or hope. Each person has his or her own unique combination of these types of tension.

The initial physiological responses that lead to tension are helpful; they are the body's way of reacting to a crisis. When we respond to a crisis, it makes sense to act quickly and forcefully. After the crisis has passed, we should let go of the physical activation and return to a more relaxed state. When that doesn't happen, the physiological activation turns into chronic tension. And chronic tension has a number of negative effects on the body.

The first of these has to do with energy depletion. It takes energy to activate the body's protective responses. When this activation persists, the increased energy drain goes on and on. The tense person feels increasingly fatigued and eventually exhausted.

Another negative effect of chronic tension is an increased chance of illness. Tight neck muscles eventually lead to tension headaches. Tight back muscles turn into low back pain. A nervous stomach becomes an ulcer or irritable bowel syndrome. A constantly racing heart turns into hypertension. Worries and fears develop into chronic anxiety. A lack of purpose in life can lead to ongoing depression.

Chronic tension also speeds up the aging process. We use up our vital resources more quickly, and without relaxation we aren't able to replenish them. Tension and stress weaken the immune system and increase the chance that an opportunistic disease or autoimmune disorder may develop. Constant overactivation of the heart and nervous system can lead to strokes, heart attacks, and death.

But the effects of tension are not just physical. Mental skills are compromised by tension. Memory becomes less efficient. Tension blocks our ability to retrieve information. It also creates a narrow, overfocused mental state that limits our experience of the world. When we are tense, we simply ignore and miss information. We aren't open to all the sights and sounds, to all the hues and textures around us.

This narrow, overfocused perception limits our problem-solving skills. We fail to perceive the multiple causes and dimensions of a problem. We often frame problems too narrowly, leading to an automatic response rather than the ability to step back, see the real dimensions of a problem, and consider the full range of solutions.

Creativity is inhibited by tension. Ability to see possibilities and new combinations is the essence of creativity. The tense, overfocused person isn't open and thus can't

Tension creates a narrow, overfocused mental state that limits our experience of the world.

express his or her natural creativity.

Tension also has a negative effect on relationships. When you are tense, it is difficult to truly listen to a partner, friend, or coworker and to understand the feelings or thoughts of others. When you are tense, you tend to be irritable and impatient. You talk from your tension rather than relax in the give-and-take of true communication. And tension inhibits the natural physiological arousal that is part of physical intimacy.

Ultimately, tension has a harmful effect on every dimension of our life. It wastes our energy and tires us out. It leads to health problems. Tension decreases mental efficiency and limits creativity. It constricts our relationships. Tension destroys our quality of life.

THE NATURE OF RELAXATION

The verb "relax" comes from the Latin *relaxare,* meaning "to loosen." From this a number of modern definitions have evolved, including: to make less tense and rigid, to relieve nervous tension, to lengthen and deactivate muscle fibers, and to seek rest and recreation. The idea of lengthening and deactivating the muscle fibers is the definition that most closely fits with the first modern work using relaxation as a therapeutic tool.

In the 1920s Dr. Edmund Jacobson pioneered the

development of a system called "Progressive Relaxation." He wrote, "By relaxation in any muscle we mean the complete absence of all contractions."[1] Conversely, tension was the contraction of the skeletal muscles. Jacobson acknowledged that it was necessary to tense the muscles for any type of coordinated physical activity. But he stressed that it was equally important to know how to totally relax the muscles.

Jacobson believed tension to be complex and potentially harmful. He noted that muscles contract at the command of the brain. If the muscles are tense, then the brain is overactive. Overactivity in the brain leads to overdrive in such internal organs as the heart, stomach, and colon. Chronic overactivity in these systems, he found, leads to a variety of health problems such as high blood pressure, irregular heartbeat, spastic colon, and upset stomach. Dr. Jacobson believed that the hectic pace and constant pressures of modern life lead inevitably to a state of chronic tension.

To remedy this problem, Progressive Relaxation trainees were taught to tense and then totally relax specific muscle groups. Jacobson noted that this system was progressive in three distinct ways. First, trainees progressively released the tension in a given muscle group. Secondly, they progressed from one muscle group to the next. Finally, with

1. Edmund Jacobson, *You Must Relax* (New York: McGraw Hill, 1962), 64.

The beneficial effects of Progressive Relaxation included rest for the skeletal muscles, a calm emotional state, improved functioning of the internal organs, and more energy.

continued practice, trainees achieved deeper and deeper levels of relaxation, for longer and longer periods.[2]

Jacobson emphasized that Progressive Relaxation was very different from mere quiet. He found that subjects sitting quietly and even sleeping would still display signs of residual tension—slight movements in the facial muscles, twitches or jumps in the fingers, continued activity in the throat, and the persistence of racing thoughts and negative emotions. The goal of Progressive Relaxation was to eliminate this residual tension and to achieve a completely relaxed state.

The beneficial effects of Progressive Relaxation included rest for the skeletal muscles, a calm emotional state, improved functioning of the internal organs, and more energy. Trainees learned to be more aware of unnecessary tension during everyday activities and to release it.

Jacobson's work in the field of relaxation established a scientific definition of relaxation, developed a systematic method for achieving relaxation, and described its beneficial effects. His original training program lasted about eighteen months. Over the years, a number of abbreviated forms of Progressive Relaxation have been developed and these are used in behavioral therapy to help people overcome specific fears.

2. Jacobson, *You Must Relax,* 94.

Another perspective on the nature of relaxation can be found in the work of Johannes Schultz and Wolfgang Luthe.[3] Beginning in the 1930s these German physicians described an autogenic state in which there was a self-induced shift to a deeply relaxed state characterized by a number of specific sensations, including feelings of warmth and heaviness in the arms and legs, a steady heart-beat, a warm abdomen, slow and easy breathing, and a cool forehead.

Schultz and Luthe developed a method called "Autogenic Training." With this method, subjects repeated mental directives describing these specific sensations, concentrating on the sensations and thereby creating the autogenic state. Subjects would say to themselves, "My arms and legs are heavy and warm," and focus on feelings of warmth and heaviness in the limbs. Once these sensations were established, subjects repeated this process with each of the other key sensations.

The autogenic state, Schultz and Luthe reported, mobilized the usually dormant normalizing and healing capabilities of the brain.[4] Subjects who created the auto-genic state on a daily basis noticed a significant reduction in fatigue and tension, fewer headaches, and greatly improved

3. J. H. Schultz and W. Luthe, *Autogenic Therapy,* vol. II (New York: Grune and Stratton, 1969), 1.

4. Schultz and Luthe, *Autogenic Therapy,* 1.

The autogenic state seemed to go beyond muscular relaxation to a complete relaxation of mind and body.

efficiency at work. With continued practice, subjects obtained dramatic relief from stress-induced disorders such as insomnia, constipation, asthma, anxiety, and phobias.

Schultz and Luthe believed autogenic training induced specific changes in control mechanisms deep in the brain. The autogenic state seemed to go beyond muscular relaxation to a complete relaxation of mind and body. They even developed phrases to be used to promote healing in specific organ systems.

Another perspective on the nature of relaxation emerged in the 1970s with the work of Dr. Herbert Benson, a professor at Harvard Medical School. He believed humans to have the capability for a unique and integrated "Relaxation Response."[5] Benson identified four elements needed to induce the Relaxation Response—a quiet environment, a comfortable position, a passive attitude, and mental repetition of a word, such as "one."[6]

Benson found that specific physiological changes occurred during the relaxation response. These included decreased oxygen consumption, decreased heart and respiratory rate, and a higher proportion of alpha brain waves. These changes represented decreased activity of the sympathetic nervous system, the part of the nervous system responsible for the fight-or-flight response. Benson

5. Herbert Benson, *The Relaxation Response* (New York: Morrow and Co., 1975), 50–52.
6. Benson, *The Relaxation Response*, 19.

believed the Relaxation Response provided a more pro-found rest and recuperation than might occur during sleep or quiet sitting.

Regular practice of the Relaxation Response, Benson discovered, led to a number of health benefits. These included reduced blood pressure and a smoother heart rate. Benson's patients reported fewer symptoms of illness, improved performance in everyday life, and feelings of satisfaction, peace, and tranquility similar to those achieved through meditation or spiritual contemplation.

These three approaches to relaxation—Progressive Relaxation, Autogenic Training, and the Relaxation Response—have a number of similarities. They all describe a self-directed method for achieving relaxation. Practiced regularly, each of these three systems is beneficial.

But there are some interesting differences. In Progressive Relaxation the emphasis is on relaxing the muscles, which then influences the brain and other organ systems. Autogenic Training focuses on relaxing the autonomic nervous system. The Relaxation Response starts by providing a mental focus; effects then filter down to the nervous system and the muscles. Is one of these approaches correct and the others wrong? Or are all three describing different aspects of relaxation?

Perhaps the key is to see relaxation as a complex response with distinct dimensions. Within each dimension

Perhaps the key is to see relaxation as a complex response with distinct dimensions.

or level, the nature of tension, the principle governing relaxation, and the methods of achieving relaxation are subtly different. The challenge is to make sense of these different techniques, to organize them, and to select the best techniques for each person.

This book is organized around five distinct dimensions of relaxation. A chapter explaining each is followed by a chapter with techniques that reduce tension on that level. This will allow the reader to understand her or his unique pattern of tension and to select those relaxation techniques most beneficial to her or him.

THE FIVE LEVELS OF RELAXATION

The Muscular Level

On the muscular level, tension is simply sustained contraction of the skeletal muscles. The experience of muscular tension is familiar to everyone. After a tough day or a demanding week, we have all felt the symptoms of muscular tension—an aching neck, tightness through the shoulders and back, a tension headache.

Muscular relaxation rids the muscles of excessive holding and tightness. The underlying principle is to direct the muscles to loosen, lengthen, and let go. There are a number of ways to accomplish this release and we will learn about them in the third chapter.

The Autonomic Level

Tension at the level of the autonomic nervous system is more complicated. This nervous system controls the inner organs and regulates heart rate, blood pressure, stomach activity, and breathing rate. The autonomic nervous system is composed of two branches. The sympathetic branch increases internal activation, while the parasympathetic branch decreases or inhibits this internal activation. Sympathetic activation prepares the body for flight or fight; the parasympathetic moves the body toward rest and relaxation. Tension at the autonomic level occurs when there is either prolonged activation or prolonged inhibition.

We experience autonomic tension inside our body. Sympathetic branch activation brings on such symptoms as heart palpitations, shortness of breath, excessive sweating, and cold, clammy hands. Parasympathetic symptoms include low energy, excessive sighing, and sluggish digestion.

The principle of relaxation at the autonomic level is balance—achieving a dynamic balance between activation and inhibition so that one feels peaceful, steady, and calm. The autogenic state described by Schultz and Luthe is autonomic relaxation. The sensations of a slow, steady heart rate, a warm abdomen, smooth breathing, and a cool forehead characterize autonomic relaxation. Chapter 5 provides practical techniques to achieve autonomic relaxation.

When we loosen the grip of negative emotions, emotions such as contentment, happiness, and joy begin to permeate our experience of life.

The Emotional Level

Tension can have a dramatic impact on your emotional state. Negative emotions such as fear, anxiety, sadness, anger, and disgust can come to dominate your outlook on life. These chronic negative emotions can lead to states of depression and helplessness. Chronic negative emotions are increasingly seen as an underlying cause of many health problems.

Emotional relaxation means letting go of chronic negative feelings. Strong feelings such as anger and fear are natural and have a protective value, but they become harmful when maintained over time. In Chapter 7 you will learn techniques to enable you to tap the energy of negative emotions and then let go of them. You will also learn how to release residues of anger and sadness stored up from the past.

Emotional relaxation also has a positive and creative side. When we loosen the grip of negative emotions, emotions such as contentment, happiness, and joy begin to permeate our experience of life. When negative emotions are dispersed, these positive, energizing, and health-giving emotions give us the experience of true emotional relaxation.

The Mental Level

Tension at the mental level involves the pattern of thoughts and the texture of perceptions. A tense mind is scattered, jumping from thought to thought, yet stuck with superficial preoccupations and obsessive thinking. Perception is restricted, narrow, and inflexible.

The experience of a tense mind is common. We may notice mental tension at the end of a long day. Our mind is revved up and scattered, preoccupied with worries and problems. When we attempt to relax, the mind keeps repeating the cycle of worries. When we try to fall asleep, our mind won't shut down. We lie there tossing and turning while our mind gallops from thought to thought.

The principle of relaxation at the mental level is an interesting combination of focus and openness. The mind is centered yet open. Many people sample mental relaxation when they engage in a hobby such as painting, building furniture, or gardening. Pleasantly absorbed in one activity, they are focused yet open and alert to possibilities. Mental relaxation might also be experienced on a long walk as we let go of our worries and become open to the sounds and sights around us. Chapter 9 presents effective techniques to directly and consciously relax the mind.

The Spiritual Level

The importance of spirituality in relaxation is reflected in the increasing use of prayer and meditation to achieve complete and deep relaxation. In fact, the most subtle tension occurs on the spiritual level. This tension is

Spiritual tension leads to feelings of alienation, isolation, and emptiness.

characterized by a lack of connection to the sacred, confusion about the purpose of life, and an absence of self-knowledge. Spiritual tension leads to feelings of alienation, isolation, and emptiness.

Spiritual tension can be alleviated when we develop a vision of the sacred, learn to know and accept ourselves, become aware of our unique inner potentials, and develop a clear sense of purpose in life. Spiritual tension is overcome when we understand nature and life around us and begin to discern the greater patterns of which our life is a part.

Chapter 11 explores a number of approaches to spiritual relaxation. We will learn to use these approaches to achieve a sense of unity, a feeling of completeness within, and a sense of connection to the world around us.

Interactions

The five levels of relaxation are not separate. They interact in many ways. Tension on one level will create tension on another level. For example, chronic anger on the emotional level might create thoughts of revenge, a churning stomach, and grinding tension in the jaws.

But these interactions between the levels can work in a positive direction. Deep muscular relaxation will calm the nervous system, decrease heart rate, smooth out breathing, and create a tranquil mind. Conversely, when we concentrate and calm the mind, we breathe more easily, we release tension in the muscles, and we feel peaceful.

The five levels of relaxation combine to form a total and integrated relaxation experience: total relaxation—a distinct capability and potential for optimal health and well-being. When we can consciously create relaxation on all five levels, we will have achieved total relaxation.

QUALITIES OF RELAXATION

What distinct qualities of relaxation are common to all five levels?

1. Relaxation Is a Learned Skill. Like many skills, relaxation is best learned through proper instruction and is mastered through persistent and attentive practice.

2. Relaxation Is a Conscious Self-Directed Skill. Many people mistakenly believe that if they sit and watch TV, read a book, or go out to dinner with friends, they will somehow relax, as if relaxation is the by-product of some pleasant activity. These pleasant activities will produce some degree of relaxation, but not enough.

The essence of deep and thorough relaxation is to

The five levels of relaxation

TENSION	RELAXATION	
Lack of pupose, alienation, isolation	Sense of the sacred, self knowledge, purpose in life	SPIRITUAL
Scattered, stuck, preoccupied mind	Focused, centered, open mind	MENTAL
Persistent, negative emotions	Letting go of negative emotions, increased positive emotions	EMOTIONAL
Excessive activation, excessive inhibition	Inner balance	AUTONOMIC
Sustained muscular contraction	Loosen, lengthen, letting go	MUSCULAR

direct attention inward, apply a systematic method, and consciously create complete relaxation. To do this, we need to learn the inner language of self-directed relaxation. At first, this may be a challenge, but with time and practice, we can become proficient in these techniques.

3. Relaxation Involves Passive Volition. The term "passive volition" comes from the field of biofeedback. It describes the process of having the intention (volition) to change an internal state yet to accomplish it without grasping for it. To relax, we should start with a clear intention and allow relaxation to happen without forcing it.

The techniques of passive volition stand in contrast to the outer world, where more effort usually brings greater results. If we want the pan to shine, we scrub it harder. If we want to earn more money, we work harder. We believe that the greater the effort, the greater the results. But striving may create tension and prevent relaxation. The key to relaxation is learning to let go.

4. Relaxation Is Individual in Nature. There is no single relaxation technique that works for everyone. People are unique in how they express tension and how they achieve relaxation. Generally, you should start on the level where you have the most tension. If you suffer from muscular tension, you should start with muscular relaxation techniques. If you have a racing nervous system, begin with autonomic relaxation techniques.

Learning style and temperament also affect your choice of relaxation techniques. If you are an auditory learner, you may prefer repeating and hearing relaxation directives; if you are a visual learner, you will respond better to images; and if you are a tactile learner, you will prefer movement and sensation.

In terms of temperament, some people prefer an emotional approach to relaxation, while others want a logical and scientific approach. Some people are most comfortable with direct, tangible techniques, while others experience relaxation as an unfolding pattern. Some need a technique that has a definite sequence and ending, while others need an ongoing process. Ultimately, each person must experiment, observe, and choose the approach that works best for them.

5. **The Effects of Relaxation Are Cumulative and Systemic.** The effects of relaxation tend to accumulate over time and to affect more and more dimensions of body, mind, and spirit.

Louise, a mother of two middle-school children who works full time, came to me because she was having frequent headaches. She also felt tired, had difficulty concentrating, and on several occasions had anxiety attacks. I taught her a combination of muscular and autonomic relaxation techniques. At first it was hard for her to relax, but after a few sessions with me, she was able to experience

The effects of relaxation tend to accumulate over time and to affect more and more dimensions of body, mind, and spirit.

a more relaxed and peaceful state. She set aside time to practice the relaxation techniques at home.

Within a few weeks, Louise noticed a decrease in the frequency and intensity of her headaches. She also noticed that she could fall asleep more easily at night, that she slept more deeply and so had more energy during the day. As she became more proficient with her relaxation, she reported that the feeling of relaxation stayed with her longer during the day. She felt less irritable, more efficient in her work, and less likely to worry. Several months later, she was pleased to be told by her doctor that her blood pressure had dropped.

After six months of practicing relaxation, Louise reported that she could achieve deep relaxation quickly. She also took mini relaxation breaks throughout the day. She was better able to consider her dreams and aspirations. Gradually her life changed as she began to do more of the things that were important to her. Among these realized priorities was the continued daily practice of relaxation.

If we analyze Louise's case, we can discern a neat progression of changes. First, she was able to stop the cycle of increasing tension that had been causing her headaches. Next she developed an awareness of relaxation in contrast to tension. As she continued to practice relaxation, this awareness deepened and the effects of relaxation began to permeate all her body systems. She slept better, had more energy, and her blood pressure dropped.

Changes then appeared on the mental and emotional levels as Louise experienced greater mental clarity and increased tranquility. She developed the capacity to respond more selectively to stressors. She could let go of anxiety and conflict. She no longer overreacted to stressful events. These changes allowed her to develop a clearer vision of her purpose in life.

This case study illustrates the cumulative and systemic effects of relaxation practice. Relaxation is not a simple intervention like taking a pill or having surgery. Relaxation requires a change in perspective. Tension did not arrive in a single day. Reversing the process by which you acquired your tension takes time and persistence.

YOUR PATTERN OF TENSION

Before turning to Chapter 2, look at the effects tension is having on your life. Review this checklist of symptoms to help you find the level(s) where you have the most tension. Then, if you want, turn to the chapter or chapters that address your unique pattern of tension. The CD that is provided features four guided practices that address different levels of relaxation.

Relaxation requires a change in perspective.

LEVEL I. MUSCULAR TENSION (Chapters 2 and 3)

Muscle spasms	*Headaches*
Neckaches	*Tight jaw*
Backaches	*Bruxism (grinding teeth)*
Tight shoulders	*Muscular tension*
Bad posture	*Nervous tics*
Leg cramps	*Tremors*

LEVEL II. AUTONOMIC NERVOUS SYSTEM TENSION (Chapters 4 and 5)

Indigestion	*Shallow or rapid breathing*
Irritable bowel	*Migraines*
Chronic constipation	*Sweaty hands*
Chronic diarrhea	*Cold hands*
High blood pressure	*Excessive sweating*
Heart palpitations	

LEVEL III. EMOTIONAL TENSION (Chapters 6 and 7)

Hostility	*Anxiety*
Irritability	*Temper outbursts*
Anger	*Fears*
Sadness	*Depression*
Crying spells	*Frustration*
Discouragement	*Phobias*
Hopelessness	

LEVEL IV. MENTAL TENSION (Chapters 8 and 9)

Distraction	*Limited perception*
Poor concentration	*Racing thoughts*
Intruding thoughts	*Confusion*
Obsessive thinking	*Worry*
Forgetfulness	*Indecision*
Preoccupation	*Weak memory*

LEVEL V. SPIRITUAL TENSION (Chapters 10 and 11)

Lack of purpose	*Alienation*
Lack of inspiration	*Loneliness*
Lack of goals and direction	*Cynicism*
Disconnection	*Lack of dreams*
Vague depression	*Boredom or ennui*

LEVEL VI. GENERAL SYMPTOMS OF TENSION

Difficulty falling asleep	*Low energy*
Restless sleep	*Paper shuffling*
Difficulty waking up	*Disorganization*
Excessive sleeping	*Decreased productivity*
Use of caffeine	*Procrastination*
Nervous eating	*Constant working*
Loss of appetite	*Weight loss/gain*
Eating more and more	*Accident proneness*
* junk food*	*Increased conflict with others*
Fatigue	

chapter two

---

muscular
tension and
relaxation

T hrough the coordinated action of groups of muscles, we are able to stand, walk, and run. With practice we can learn to dance, to do somersaults, to leap into the air and land with perfect balance. As infants we struggle to hold on to a rattle or a bottle, but as we grow up, we can learn to write, to sew, to draw, and even to perform microsurgery. We can use our muscles to move gracefully through life, to work, to love, to create works of art, and to express our feelings.

All of these constructive activities are accomplished when our brain and muscles work smoothly together, selectively initiating and then releasing muscular activity. But all too often this smooth teamwork of brain and muscles breaks down. The muscles remain activated, the brain keeps sending commands to activate the muscles, and a cycle of muscular tension is created. Our movements become restricted, our posture unbalanced. Eventually this tension leads to headaches, back aches, and neck pain.

To avoid these problems, we need to understand how the muscles work and what we can do to relax our muscles. The word "muscle" comes from the Latin word *musculus,* which means "mouse." Perhaps the ancients saw a similarity between the shape of certain muscles and the form of a mouse. We now define "muscle" as fibrous tissue that contracts when stimulated and moves the limbs, trunk, and internal organs.

The motor neuron emerges from the spinal cord and branches out at its end to connect with a number of individual muscle fibers.

Actually, there are three types of muscle. *Cardiac muscles* in the heart create the rhythmic contractions that pump the blood through the body. *Smooth muscles* are found in internal organs such as the stomach, intestines, uterus, blood vessels, and bladder. The contraction of these muscles in the stomach and intestines moves food through the digestive system. Our concern is the *skeletal muscles* that connect to the bones and cross the joints and make up 40 to 50 percent of our body weight. The skeletal muscles give us the capability to stand and move.

Large muscles like the biceps are made up of numerous muscle fibers. The biceps narrow at the ends, forming tough fibrous tendons which attach to the bones. The fleshy belly of the muscle is wrapped in a fibrous covering which contains it and separates it from surrounding tissue. Muscles are richly nourished by capillaries which provide a constant supply of glucose and oxygen when the muscles are in movement.

The most important functional aspect of the muscles is the motor unit. This refers to a small group of muscle fibers controlled by a single nerve known as a motor neuron. The motor neuron emerges from the spinal cord and branches out at its end to connect with a number of muscle fibers. The activation of a single motor neuron causes these fibers to contract. Within a major muscle such as the biceps, motor units fire in a synchronous pattern that adds up to a smooth contraction. When greater effort is required, more motor units are activated.

The activation of the motor units is controlled by a part of the brain called the *sensory motor cortex*. This part of the brain orchestrates complex movements like walking, lifting, or grasping. Such movements demand coordination and efficiency. As infants, we have difficulty with these coordinated movements. But as we grow up, the brain and muscles learn to work together smoothly. In the case of athletes, artists, and musicians, this coordination may develop to astounding levels of proficiency.

The sensory motor cortex not only sends motor signals out to activate the muscles, it also receives sensory information coming in from the muscles. When any muscle contracts, information on the strength of that contraction is sent back to the brain. Similarly, when a muscle tires or is in pain, this information is sent back. If you close your eyes and tighten the muscles in your right hand, you can notice the lines of communication between your brain and your muscles.

Tension is created when there is a breakdown in the smooth communication and teamwork between muscles and brain. There may be too many signals going out from the brain contracting muscles, and too little information registering in the brain on the amount of contraction.

If you close your eyes and tighten the muscles in your right hand, you can notice the lines of communication between your brain and your muscles.

The combination of sustained contraction and limited awareness creates a cycle of ever increasing tension.

Muscular relaxation is based on conscious awareness of the amount of tension in the muscles, coupled with the ability to directly release unneeded and excessive muscular activation. These two skills, conscious awareness and direct control, can be used to break the cycle of tension and restore the muscular system to a state of balance. But before we learn specific relaxation techniques, we need to understand the causes of chronic muscular tension.

PATTERNS OF TENSION

Constant, repetitive use of certain muscles is one major cause of muscular tension. This happens when we repeat a certain posture or movement over and over. For example, many people do a great deal of sitting, creating a postural habit of leaning forward, flexing the lower back and upper back and hyperextending the neck.

All of this sitting and flexing forward creates a specific and fairly common imbalance. Over months and years, this pattern accumulates tension in the neck and the back. The muscles begin to adapt and shorten, locking us into a pattern of tension. Only when the tension reaches a level where we have a throbbing headache or painfully sore back do we realize that something is wrong. Even then we are likely to ignore this information by taking pain relievers to cover up the symptoms.

There are many other instances where repeated use leads to tension. Some people stare at a computer screen all day. Not only do they lean forward, but often they tighten the muscles around their eyes to focus on the screen. Keyboarding all day long can lead to patterns of tension in the hands and wrists as well as in the neck and face. Many assembly jobs involve repetitive patterns of reaching, lifting, and carrying that can lead to increasingly common conditions such as tendonitis and carpal tunnel syndrome.

In all of these activities, our conscious awareness is directed to the task at hand and away from our posture. We are focusing so intently on the task that the feedback from tension in our muscles doesn't register.

Overuse of muscles is another behavioral pattern that contributes to chronic tension. Many people rush from dawn until midnight. The day begins with the jarring ring of the alarm clock. Then the morning scramble starts, rushing to get showered and dressed, herding the kids to breakfast and the school bus, and jumping into the car to do battle with the other commuters. Then there is the full day of work with all of its hurrying, sitting, talking, thinking, and effort. Another battle with traffic sets the stage for home and the challenges of dinner, kids' activities, community meetings, classes, and home projects.

Keyboarding all day long can lead to patterns of tension in the hands and wrists as well as in the neck and face.

All day long we have been relentlessly firing up the muscles. Each confrontation, each challenge, each struggle causes a little more tightness in the shoulders, neck, back, and jaw. So it is no wonder that when we finally collapse into bed, we just can't relax and drift off to sleep. Too much tension has accumulated through the day. And even if we do finally fall asleep, our residual tension causes a restless, fitful sleep. We wake tired the next morning to start the day with a backlog of tension carried over from the day before.

Strong negative emotions such as fear and anger can cause muscular tension. If we feel scared, we are either paralyzed with fear or are ready to run. If we feel rage, we tighten our arms, close our hands into fists, clench our jaws, and are ready to hit and even bite. With anxiety, we feel on edge, our muscles tight and shaky. When we feel disgust, we turn up our noses and turn our heads away. When we are sad, we frown and tighten the muscles around our eyes.

If we experience strong emotions during the day, our muscles are on alert and ready to move. But most of the time our emotions and the associated impetus for movement are not expressed. We force a smile over unresolved anger. We paint a veneer of calmness over our fear, anxiety, and worry. The underlying emotions and the muscular activation remain and turn into tension.

Strong negative emotions such as fear and anger can cause muscular tension.

This tension can remain with us for a long time. Some psychotherapists maintain that the emotional traumas and unresolved conflicts from childhood are embedded in patterns of muscular tension in a self-perpetuating cycle. The person who feels sad and lonely stretches his head and torso forward as if he is reaching out for nurturing. But this body language puts others off and they draw back. Feeling even more sad and lonely, the rejected person leans a little more forward, and the cycle of emotionally based tension is reinforced.

Similar patterns of body language occur for other emotions. A person gripped by fear arouses fear in others. The person holding onto anger provokes defensiveness and anger. An anxious, tense person makes other people nervous.

These patterns of muscular tension not only shape our emotional and mental experience, but create filters that affect our perception of the world. Only with complete muscular relaxation can we get beyond these self-defeating circuits to experience life in a spontaneous and direct manner.

THE EFFECTS OF MUSCULAR TENSION

Normally, when the muscles relax, blood flow increases, the muscle fibers receive crucial nutrients, and the waste

Every action has
an added element
of struggle when
we have to work
around tension.

products of cellular metabolism are carried away. This process of nourishment and cleansing allows the muscles to be healthy and to function smoothly.

When the muscles remain tense, this process is disrupted. Toxins build up in the muscles, and the muscle cells don't receive the nutrients they need. Over time, the overall health of the muscles declines. As a result, the muscles can't respond as strongly and can't sustain effort during times of peak demand. The muscles also become much more vulnerable to aches, stiffness, and spasm.

A second effect of muscular tension is gradual restriction of movement and flexibility. When our muscles are tensed, we move less freely; a person might take a walk, but his or her neck and shoulder muscles remain tight. These tense muscles don't get the beneficial stretching and loosening that the walking could provide.

Patterns of muscular tension also interfere with the efficiency of body movement. When we walk, we have to overcome the burden created by tension in our legs, back, and neck. Every action has an added element of struggle when we have to work around tension. This struggle causes tension in surrounding muscles and puts more stress on the heart and other organs.

Normally, the muscles send sensory information back to the brain regarding the level of tension in the muscles, their location in space, and any sensations of discomfort.

With chronic tension, we lose awareness of this sensory information. We become like the person who lives next to an interstate highway but no longer hears the traffic. Yet the constant din creates tension just as the continuing signals of tension and discomfort in the nervous system lead to even more stress.

PRINCIPLES OF MUSCULAR RELAXATION

The most important dimension of learning muscular relaxation is reestablishment of awareness of the control and information pathways that run the muscles, so that we can learn how to selectively reduce muscular activation. Only then can we begin to achieve complete relaxation.

> Align your body so that you can picture a straight line going from your forehead... and ending between your feet and toes.

The muscular relaxation techniques offered in this book are designed to systematically develop this awareness and control. Once you have mastered the beginning steps of conscious self-directed relaxation, you can progress to deeper and more profound levels of relaxation.

RELAXATION BASICS

The best position for relaxation is to lie on your back on a carpeted floor. Bring your legs together and your arms alongside your body. Align your body so that you can picture a straight line going from your forehead, over your nose, to your chin, to the middle of your chest, to your navel, between your knees, to end between your feet and toes. Then move your legs so that each knee is six to eight inches away from that center line. Move your arms away from your body so there is about six to eight inches between your elbow and the side of your body, with your palms facing up.

The posture is called Shavasana in the tradition of hatha yoga. Shavasana means "corpse pose," the idea being that when you practice this relaxation posture, you shed your tense, uptight, stressed-out body to be reborn with a body relaxed, refreshed, and renewed.

In Shavasana or any posture used for relaxation, the most important thing is to be comfortable and pain free. You may be more comfortable with a small pillow under your neck or under your knees. If you have mobility problems that preclude lying on the floor, then a comfortable chair can be used. Stretching out on a bed is usually not a good idea because relaxation practice demands that you maintain alertness and conscious control.

What else do you need? The first thing is a quiet room where you will be reasonably free of interruptions. Because a relaxed state tends to lower body temperatures, you may want to wear something that will keep you warm. Loose, comfortable clothing is best. Remove your belt, watch, glasses, contact lenses, or any constricting items. Avoid any breeze or draft that might chill you, and make sure the room isn't so warm as to make you sleepy.

There is no required time of day to practice relaxation. Relaxation early in the morning can help to set the tone for the day. Relaxation in the middle of the day can help to restore a sense of calmness and prevent the accumulation of tension. Relaxation after work is an ideal way to wind down. And a session of relaxation before bedtime can help prepare you for a deep and restful sleep. Find a time that fits your schedule. When you practice is not nearly as important as having a regular daily practice.

Not everyone is going to be immediately comfortable with the basic relaxation posture or the process of relaxation. If you are accustomed to high levels of tension, you may initially feel anxious during relaxation practice. If you have this response, you may be more comfortable in a position known as the "crocodile pose," in which you lie on your stomach, cross your arms, and rest your forehead on your arms, spreading your feet twelve to eighteen inches apart. This posture often feels more protected and safe.

Now you are ready to learn systematic relaxation techniques. These techniques will emphasize the principles of increasing your inner awareness and developing conscious control over your muscles.

When you practice is not nearly as important as having a regular daily practice.

chapter three

Level I:
muscular relaxation
techniques

T here are two categories of muscular relaxation techniques: *direct* and *indirect*. The direct techniques are based on consciously and directly decreasing the level of activation in the muscles. These techniques help to develop precise awareness and control of muscle activation. This chapter presents four direct techniques. With indirect techniques, relaxation is created as a by-product of some other activity. A vigorous workout that leaves you tired but pleasantly relaxed is one good example of an indirect approach to relaxation.

DIRECT METHODS OF RELAXATION

Systematic Tense-Release Relaxation

The Systematic Tense-Release Relaxation (STRR) technique involves selectively contracting and then relaxing specific muscles throughout the body. For each muscle, you follow a specific set of steps. First, you contract the muscle, creating noticeable tension in that muscle. Focus on the sensations of tension in that muscle. Then gradually release the tension. Continue to let go and loosen the muscle until it is more relaxed than when you started. Notice the sensations of relaxation in that muscle.

As you progress through the body's major muscle groups, you are creating a state of complete relaxation. You are learning to recognize the sensations of tension and

The Systematic Tense-Release Relaxation (STRR) technique involves selectively contracting and then relaxing specific muscles throughout the body.

relaxation, and discovering how to work with the control centers in your brain that activate and relax muscles.

You can read the procedure for Systematic Tense-Release Relaxation below, memorize it, and then follow the steps. Or you can read the steps onto a tape and then play it back and follow the directions.

The pace of STRR should be brisk to keep it an active, conscious process. Contract each muscle for a count of five seconds, and release for five to ten seconds. As you become experienced in STRR, you may find it comfortable to inhale with the contraction and exhale with the release.

Bring your attention to your right hand. Make a fist and hold the tension, noticing the sensations.

the practice

- Assume the Shavasana relaxation pose. Take several easy, smooth breaths and feel the floor support you.
- Bring your attention to your right hand. Make a fist and hold the tension, noticing the sensations. Then slowly release the tension. Let go and loosen the fingers. Keep letting go, and notice the sensations that go with loosening the muscles.
  - Stretch your right hand up and back toward the top of your lower arm. Notice the tension in the top of your lower arm, hold it, and release. Let those

muscles loosen and lengthen underneath the skin. Notice the sensations.

- Bend your right hand toward the inside of the wrist. Notice the tension on the inside of the lower arm, hold it, and then slowly release. Let the muscles loosen and lengthen. Notice the experience of loosening the muscles in your lower right arm.

- Straighten your right arm at the elbow and feel tension in the triceps, the muscles underneath your upper arm. Hold and feel the tightness. Now slowly let go.

- Bend your right arm at the elbow, bringing your hand toward your shoulder, and feel the tightening in the biceps. Hold the tension and then let go. Keep on releasing. Notice the sensations that accompany loosening and deactivating the muscles.

- Now make a fist with your left hand, tighten it, and feel the tension. Then let go, release and loosen the fingers. Let them unfold and lengthen. Notice the sensations.

- Now stretch your left hand back, feel the tension on the top of the lower arm. Hold it, and release. Keep on releasing.

- Curl your fingers forward, tightening the muscles on the bottom of the left forearm. Feel the tension. Release it and notice the sensation of lengthening and

Bend your right arm at the elbow, bringing your hand toward your shoulder, and feel the tightening in the biceps.

Feel the tension in your foot. Then release, loosen the toes, and lengthen the muscles under the skin.

softening those muscles.

- Straighten your left arm at the elbow, tensing the left triceps. Hold it, and then let go. Keep on letting go. Feel the muscle loosening.
- Bend your left arm at the elbow, bringing your hand to your shoulder, and feel the tightness in the biceps. Hold the tension for a few seconds, and then let go. Let the arm come back down to the floor. Keep on letting go.
  - Now direct your awareness to your right foot. Curl the toes of that foot. Feel the tension in your foot. Then release, loosen the toes, and lengthen the muscles under the skin.
  - Point your right foot out away from the body. Be aware of the tension in the muscles along the outside of your lower leg. Hold the tension, then let go. Notice the experience of releasing the tension.
  - Stretch your right foot back toward your body and feel the tension in the calf muscle. Hold the tightness, notice the sensation, then let go and keep on letting go. Observe the sensations of releasing and relaxing.
- Straighten your right leg at the knee and feel the tension in the quadriceps muscles on top of your right thigh. Hold the tension, release, and keep on releasing, lengthening and softening the muscles in the upper leg.

- Bend your right knee and bring your leg up toward your body, knee over your abdomen. Feel the tightness inside your right upper leg. Hold the tension, then release and let your leg come back down. Direct the muscles to keep on releasing.
- Now curl the toes of your left foot. Hold the tension and feel the activation in the muscles. Then release and be aware of the lengthening and softening of the muscles.
- Point your left foot out away from your body. Feel the tension in the muscles along the outside of your lower leg. Release the tension and keep on letting go.
- Bend your left foot back toward your body and be aware of the tension in your calf muscle. Notice the sensation of tension, then release that holding. Loosen and lengthen the calf muscle. Observe the sensations of releasing the muscle in your calf.
- Straighten your left leg and feel the tension in the left quadriceps. Hold it, and then release. Keep on releasing, and notice the sensations as you decrease activity in the muscle.
- Bend your left leg at the knee, bringing the knee up over your abdomen, and feel the tightness inside your thigh. Now release that holding, let your leg come back down. Continue to let go in your upper leg.
- Now bring your awareness to the muscles of your face.

Bend your left leg at the knee, bringing the knee up over your abdomen, and feel the tightness inside your thigh.

Lift your eyebrows and wrinkle your forehead. Observe the sensations of tightness across the forehead. Hold it, and then release. Repeat two times. Completely release the muscles across the forehead. Feel the sensation of smoothing the forehead.

- Squint your eyes shut. Feel the tension in all the tiny muscles around your eyes. Then let go and direct those muscles to loosen beneath the skin. Repeat this two times. Keep on letting go around the eyes. Notice the feeling as you loosen all the muscles around your eyes.
- Clench your teeth and tighten your jaw muscles. Feel that tension, hold it, then release and soften the jaw muscles. Repeat this twice. Study the feeling that comes with softening any holding in the jaw muscles.
- Push your lips up toward your nose. Hold, and then release. Repeat this two times. Then release the muscles around the lips.

Notice the feelings and sensations of decreasing the activity in the facial muscles.

- Stretch your mouth open as far as it can go. Hold that tension, and then release. Repeat this two times. Then let go through the entire lower face and jaw. Notice the feelings and sensations of decreasing the activity in the facial muscles.
- Lift your head a few inches off the floor, tightening the muscles on the front of the neck. Slowly turn your head to the right, tightening the muscles on the right side of

the neck. Then turn your head to the left, tightening the muscles on the left side of the neck. Bring your head back to the center and let it ease to the floor. Let all the muscles in the neck release, lengthen, and soften beneath the skin. Repeat this two times.

- Bring your shoulders forward, and release. Lift your shoulders toward your head, and let go. Pull your shoulders back, then release. Let all of the holding out of the shoulders. Repeat this two times. Then let go completely in the shoulders.

- Tighten the muscles across your abdomen. Hold the tension and feel it. Then release, decreasing the activity in the abdominal muscles. Notice the experience of softening those muscles.

- Tighten your lower back, flattening it against the floor. Hold the tension, and release. Continue to let go.

- Tighten up your buttocks. Hold the tension, and then release it.

- Take several easy, smooth breaths.

- Step by step, bring your awareness back through all the muscles you have been releasing, and just let go a little more. Let go of any last residual tension. Soften and lengthen the muscles in the feet, lower legs, upper legs, pelvis and hips, stomach, lower back, chest, upper back, shoulders, upper arms, lower arms, hands, neck, lips, jaw, eyes, and forehead. Be aware of letting the muscles relax

all over your body. Enjoy the state of relaxation and quiet.
• After a few minutes of this quiet, take a few deeper breaths, move your fingers and toes, and take a long, lazy stretch, reaching your arms above you. When you are ready, comfortably come to a sitting position. Resume the day's activities, keeping a feeling of relaxation.

This technique is very helpful for people who suffer from tension headaches, insomnia, or any muscular pain. STRR is a good technique for beginners because it is active and systematic. Daily practice of this method can significantly decrease anxiety and stress.

Differential Relaxation

In Differential Relaxation, you activate the muscles on one side of the body while keeping muscles on the other side of the body loose and passive. As you focus on the difference between the active and passive muscles, you become more aware of the difference between tension and relaxation. For example, as you tighten the muscles in the right arm, you pay attention to keeping the muscles in the left arm relaxed.

The key terms with this method are "active" and "passive." When you make one set of muscles active, you keep the other set passive. This helps you become more attuned to the sensations of tension and relaxation. With practice, you can refine your ability to identify the control systems in your brain that allow you to activate and relax muscles selectively throughout the body.

Differential Relaxation greatly increases your inner awareness and is a very effective relaxation technique. The CD accompanying this book contains a guided practice with Differential Relaxation. Remember to hold each contraction for five to ten seconds and to release for ten to twenty seconds.

Guided Relaxation

Guided Relaxation involves a shift away from physically tensing and releasing muscles to a more mentally guided approach. With this technique, you bring your attention to specific muscles and direct those muscles to relax.

This more subtle technique works best after you have experience with Systematic Tense-Release Relaxation or Differential Relaxation. You must have a good sense of where the muscles are, how they feel when tense, and how to direct them to relax. You have to be able to sustain your attention on each muscle group. Properly practiced, this technique can lead to deep levels of relaxation.

As with the other methods, you can memorize these instructions and use them, or tape-record and listen to them. This technique can be used independently or following Systematic Tense-Release Relaxation or Differential Relaxation. You should spend about ten to twenty seconds

Guided Relaxation works best after you have experience with Systematic Tense-Release Relaxation or Differential Relaxation.

focusing on each muscle group, locating it, noticing any tension, and directing the muscle to release.

the
practice

- Assume the Shavasana relaxation posture. Take several deep breaths, and then let your breathing settle into a smooth rhythm. Let go and let the floor support you.
  - Bring your full attention to your right foot. Notice any tension on the top of the foot, bottom of the foot, or in the toes. Then release, lengthening and softening the muscles in the foot.
  - Now bring your awareness to your right lower leg. Notice any holding or tightness in the calf or shin. Study that tension, then release it, letting go in the lower leg.
- Bring your attention to the muscles in the right upper leg, to the quadriceps on top of the leg, the thigh muscles, and the muscles at the back of the leg. Notice any residual tension in these muscles. Then direct the muscles in the upper leg to loosen and lengthen. Notice the sensation of the muscles becoming passive.
- Now bring your awareness to the left foot. Consider the muscles in the toes, across the top of the foot, and on the

Bring your full attention to your right foot. Notice any tension on the top of the foot, bottom of the foot, or in the toes.

bottom of the foot. Check for any holding in these muscles. Then just soften them, guiding the muscles to a passive, loose state.

- Pay attention to the lower left leg. Bring your awareness first to the calf muscle, then to the shin. Notice the amount of holding and tension in these muscles. Direct the muscles to loosen and lengthen. Notice the sensation as the muscles relax.

- Move your awareness to your left upper leg, to the quadriceps on top of the leg, the thigh muscles, and the muscles at the back of the leg. Notice any tension or holding in these muscles. Gradually guide the muscles to lengthen and loosen. Decrease the activity and feel the sensation of releasing.

- Now bring your attention to your buttocks. Notice any tension or holding in those muscles. Then just direct them to go passive. Notice the sensation of relaxing these muscles.

- Direct your awareness to your pelvic region. Notice the layers of muscles. Detect any levels of tension, then release the holding. Let the muscles lengthen.

- Now bring your full attention to your lower back. Notice any tension in this area. Study the feeling that this tension creates. Then with each exhalation, let go in the lower back. Soften and loosen the

Bring your full attention to your lower back. Notice any tension in this area.

muscles, open them. Notice the sensations that accompany relaxing these muscles.

- Become aware of the muscles along the spinal column from the lower back up to the neck. Feel the tightness in these muscles. Command the muscles to loosen and lengthen. Soften those muscles, and notice the sensation of relaxation along your spine.

Bring your awareness to the abdominal muscles. Notice the tension across the stomach.

- Attend to the muscles around your shoulder blades. Feel the degree of holding in these muscles. Notice how that holding feels, the sensations of that tension. Direct those muscles to soften, lengthen, and loosen. Notice the shift to a more relaxed condition in these muscles.

- Now bring your awareness to the abdominal muscles. Notice the tension across the stomach. With each exhalation, release that tension. Feel the muscles soften and loosen. Notice how your whole body becomes more relaxed as you let go across your abdomen.

- Now focus on the muscles across the chest, the pectoral muscles. Notice the tension in these muscles. With each exhalation, release the holding in them. Lengthen and soften them beneath the skin.

- Now bring your awareness to the shoulders. Notice the holding and tension lodged in the shoulders. Feel the sensations that go with that tension. Let go in your shoulders. Let them drop. Release the holding from the front and back of the shoulders. Lengthen and soften the muscles. Feel the shift in your shoulders and throughout your body as you release the shoulders. Notice the sensations of relaxation.

• Bring your awareness to your right upper arm, to the triceps and the biceps. Notice any residual tension in the upper arm and notice the feelings associated with that slight tension. Now direct the muscles in the upper right arm to release, to lengthen and soften. Notice how it feels when the muscles in the upper arm relax.

• Move your attention to your lower right arm and notice the muscles on top of and underneath the lower right arm. Check for residual tension in those muscles. Then let go of tension, release, and smooth the muscles. Be aware of the sensation of relaxation in your lower arm.

• Now bring your awareness to your right hand and consider the muscles on top of the hand, in the palm, and out along the fingers. Start to notice the lingering tension in the muscles of the right hand. Then loosen those muscles, let go, and release any holding in the right hand and fingers. Notice the shift in the right hand and throughout the body when you release the muscles in your right hand and fingers.

• Direct your awareness to the left upper arm, the biceps and triceps. Scan those muscles to

Bring your awareness to your right hand and consider the muscles on top of the hand, in the palm, and out along the fingers.

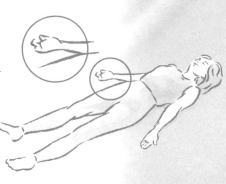

detect the amount of residual tension. Observe the sensations associated with that tension. Watch those sensations change as you consciously direct the muscles to soften and loosen. Let go and lengthen the muscles in your left upper arm.

- Move your awareness down to the left lower arm, to the muscles on top of the arm and underneath the lower arm. Study the muscles and notice any remaining tension. Direct those muscles to lengthen and soften. Let go.

- Guide your attention to your left hand, the muscles across the palm, the top of the hand, and in the fingers. Notice any subtle residual tension lingering in the left hand. Let go. Direct the muscles in the left hand to loosen, lengthen, and soften. Notice the subtle shift in consciousness as you completely relax your left hand.

- Direct your attention to the back of the neck. Notice the tension lodged there. Direct those muscles to loosen and soften. Let go, and feel the sensations that go with releasing the neck muscles.

- Now move your awareness up to the back of the head. Be aware of any tension at the back of your head. Direct the muscles to soften and release. Notice the shift that occurs with loosening those muscles.

- Bring your awareness to the forehead. Feel any holding or tightness across the forehead. Notice the constriction that goes with that holding. Loosen those muscles, make the forehead smooth, and feel the freedom that goes with relaxed muscles across the forehead. Feel your cares ease away as you smooth out the forehead.

- Bring your attention to the tiny muscles around the eyes. Feel any tightness that has collected in the eye muscles. Little by little, release the holding around the eyes, smooth the muscles around your eyes. Notice the feelings that go with relaxing your eye muscles.

- Guide your awareness to the jaw muscles. Feel the tightness held there. Notice how the tension feels. Then release that unneeded tension, drop the holding, loosen the muscles. Notice the sensation of relaxation in the jaw muscles.

- Direct your awareness to the muscles around the lips and 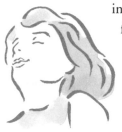 in the lower face, the muscles that can hold a frown. Notice any patterns of holding and tightness. Feel the sensations of that holding. Then release that tension, loosen the muscles, soften them. Feel a natural, subtle smile form as you relax your lips and lower face.

Feel a natural, subtle smile form as you relax your lips and lower face.

- Now guide your awareness to your breathing. Let your breaths be easy and smooth. Scan your entire body for any lingering tension and release that holding. Let your

Bring your arms up over your head and take a nice, long stretch.

awareness rest on your breathing for a while.

• When you are ready, let a sense of activity gradually return to your limbs. Take a few deeper breaths and wiggle the fingers and toes. Bring your arms up over your head and take a nice, long stretch. Sit up when you are ready, and resume the activities of your day, keeping a feeling of relaxation and peacefulness.

Rotation of Consciousness

Rotation of Consciousness is the most subtle of the direct relaxation techniques for muscular relaxation. You simply guide your awareness through specific points on your body. Because tension in a muscle is caused by a lack of awareness, when you bring full awareness to that muscle, relaxation occurs spontaneously. You don't have to do anything like tensing or releasing, you just have to move your full awareness through specific points in your body.

This technique introduces the concept of non-doing or non-effort. In the three previous techniques, you needed to do something in order to relax. But using effort to relax is a bit of a paradox. The effort itself creates some degree of tension. With this method there is no effort, just the systematic flow of awareness from one part of the body to another. This approach can create a most profound state of relaxation.

CHAPTER THREE

To practice this technique, think the name of a part of the body and focus your full awareness on that part. For example, you might think or say inwardly "right index finger" and bring your full awareness to the right index finger. Keep your awareness there for five seconds, then move to the next point.

As with the methods described above, you can memorize and then follow the instructions, or record them on a tape and listen to them.

the practice

- Assume the Shavasana relaxation pose. Take several deep breaths, then let your breathing become smooth and easy.
- Bring your awareness to the right hand. Now attend to the right thumb, right index finger, right middle finger, right ring finger, right little finger, right palm, back of the right hand, right wrist, top of the right lower arm, underneath the lower right arm, right elbow, right biceps, right triceps, right shoulder, right armpit, right side of the torso, right waist, right hip, right thigh, right knee, right calf, right shin, right ankle, right heel, sole of the right foot, top of the right foot, right big toe, right second toe, right middle toe, right fourth toe, right little toe.

Bring your awareness to your left hand. Focus your awareness on the left thumb, left index finger, left middle finger, left ring finger, and left little finger.

- Now bring your awareness to your left hand. Focus your awareness on the left thumb, left index finger, left middle finger, left ring finger, and left little finger. Now move your awareness to the left palm, back of the left hand, left wrist, top of the left lower arm, underneath the left lower arm, left elbow, left biceps, left triceps, left shoulder, left armpit, left side of the torso, left waist, left hip, left thigh, left knee, left calf, left shin, and left ankle. Guide your awareness to the heel of the left foot, the sole of the left foot, the top of the left foot, the left big toe, left second toe, left middle toe, left fourth toe, and the left little toe.
- Now bring your awareness to the back of the neck, to the right shoulder blade, the left shoulder blade, along the spinal column, the lower back, the right buttock, and the left buttock.
- Bring your awareness to the top of your head, to the forehead, right temple, left temple, right eye, left eye, the spot between the two eyebrows, right cheek, left cheek, right jaw, left jaw, lips, chin, neck, right side of the chest, left side of the chest, right side of the abdomen, left side of the abdomen, right side of the pelvis, and left side of the pelvis.
- Bring your attention to the whole right arm; the whole left arm; both arms; the whole right leg; the whole left

leg; both legs; the whole back, including the neck, shoulder blades, spine, lower back, and buttocks; and the whole front of the body, including the chest, abdomen, and pelvis. Then bring your awareness to the whole body.

- Bring your attention to your breath. Breathe evenly and smoothly. Enjoy the deep, rejuvenating quiet of relaxation. When you are ready, slowly and gently bring activity back to the fingers and feet, to the arms and legs, by moving them slightly. Bring your hands up over your head and take a long, easy stretch. Then when you are ready, get up and resume the activity of the day. Carry the deep peace of relaxation with you.

INDIRECT MUSCULAR RELAXATION TECHNIQUES

Muscular tension can be thought of as an activity potential trapped in the muscle fibers. When we are exposed to stressors throughout the day, we activate the muscles in two basic and primitive ways: to fight or to flee. When these impulses are not expressed, they accumulate as tension in the muscles.

One way to release this tension is to perform exercise similar to fighting or fleeing. This type of exercise brings these trapped impulses to full expression. Then we are able to relax fully.

When we are exposed to stressors throughout the day, we activate the muscles in two basic and primitive ways: to fight or to flee.

Fleeing exercises include running, walking, swimming, biking, cross-country skiing, ice skating, roller skating, and roller blading. Aerobics can be included in this category. Fleeing-type exercise should be performed three to seven times a week to be effective.

Keep in mind that this exercise is not a training regimen, but a means of reducing stress and expressing trapped muscular tension. Make the activity pleasurable by exercising in the fresh air with inspiring scenery or in a pleasing indoor environment. An overly competitive approach will just add to your tension and stress.

Exercises that express the trapped impulse to fight typically involve some element of struggle. Weight lifting is one example. The exertion required to lift heavier amounts for more repetitions helps to express the energy of struggle. Again, the idea is not to lift extremely heavy weights, but to find weights that will test your strength, work on a variety of muscles, and express trapped fighting tension.

Many competitive sports allow for socially approved expression of aggression. Tennis, squash, racquetball, and even badminton involve a clear element of struggle. After a good match, many people feel more relaxed. Cultivating the right attitude when playing these sports—playing hard, striving but keeping a sense of enjoyment—will enhance the relaxation effect.

Martial arts provide another approach to channeling

and expressing fighting energy. The routines or *katas* of karate, with their punching, kicking, and blocking, provide a direct expression of aggression in a disciplined manner.

Stretching exercises are another way to achieve muscular relaxation. Stretching exercises gradually and gently relieve stored-up muscle tension. Hatha yoga is a complete system containing postures *(asanas)* designed to stretch muscles throughout the body.

The manner of practicing these postures is unique. You stretch into the posture until you begin to experience some tightness and resistance. At that point you breathe, relax, and ease ever so gently farther into the posture. This gentle stretching approach releases patterns of holding and tension, gradually opening and lengthening tense muscles. With regular practice, the stiffest person can become looser and more flexible.

There are a number of books and videos that provide hatha yoga instruction. Learning basic yoga postures and practicing them daily can be a very useful way to decrease muscular tension. This form of exercise is not well understood in Western culture where the prevailing belief is that exercise must be rigorous and even painful if it is to bring results. With the Hatha Yoga postures, the more focus, care, and gentleness you bring to exercise, the better the results.

GUIDELINES FOR PRACTICE

We have explored a number of techniques for achieving muscular relaxation. You should practice one of the direct relaxation techniques at least once a day and if possible, twice. Active exercise can be performed three to five times a week. Stretching exercises should be done five to seven times a week.

While muscular relaxation balances the nervous system, calms the mind, creates emotional serenity, and provides a greater sense of clarity and purpose in life, there are other relaxation methods that address these levels more directly. In the next two chapters, we will explore the nature of the autonomic nervous system and learn relaxation techniques for this level.

chapter four

---

tension within

the autonomic

nervous system

We all know the inner experience of stress. In a moment of danger or at a time when we had to perform under pressure, we have all felt a pounding heart, gasping shallow breaths, a dry mouth, cold clammy hands, nervous sweating, knots in the stomach, and a shaky voice.

All of these intense and involuntary physical changes are controlled by the autonomic nervous system. The term "autonomic" describes the automatic nature of this activation. We don't have to decide to increase our heart rate, shut down our digestion, constrict the blood vessels in our hands, or breathe rapidly. In an instant all of these organ systems respond to support fighting or fleeing.

When the danger is past, this inner mobilization of our nervous system should subside. But all too often this inner stress response is sustained. The heart keeps on beating rapidly, blood pressure rises, and stress chemicals flow through the bloodstream. The resulting chronic autonomic stress can be damaging and ultimately lethal.

We may feel we have no way to control and regulate this inner stress response. Consequently, we resort to mechanistic methods to reduce autonomic tension and its effects. We take tranquilizers to calm our nerves. We take medication to reduce blood pressure and slow the heartbeat. We have a drink to help us relax. We swallow antacids for indigestion. These remedies provide temporary relief, but they do not address the underlying problem of chronic autonomic tension.

With effective
autonomic relaxation
we can significantly
reduce the stress on
our heart, digestive
system, and
endocrine system
and enhance the
function of our
immune system.

Self-directed relaxation of the ANS is possible. But the methods are qualitatively different from those of muscular relaxation. With the muscles, we used the voluntary nervous system and directly commanded the muscles to become active or passive. Relaxation at the autonomic level means acquiring a whole new set of skills. We need to learn to access the more indirect pathways that control the ANS. We need to learn to calm the heartbeat, regulate the breath, and quiet the autonomic turbulence within.

The benefits are tremendous. With effective autonomic relaxation we can significantly reduce the stress on our heart, digestive system, and endocrine system and enhance the function of our immune system. We have more energy and vitality. When we are more in control of our body, we are more in control of our life.

THE AUTONOMIC NERVOUS SYSTEM

The autonomic nervous system has two branches: sympathetic and parasympathetic. The sympathetic branch activates the body for fight or flight. The parasympathetic branch moves the body into a state designed for rest and housekeeping.

The nerves of the sympathetic branch leave the spinal column at various points from the neck down to the lower back, as seen in figure 1. These fibers travel to the heart, bronchi, stomach, adrenal gland, kidneys, intestine, and anal sphincter. Sympathetic nerves also reach the sweat glands and the blood vessels in the periphery of the body. Sympathetic nerves also affect the piloerector muscles that make the hair on our arms and at the back of our neck stand up when we are afraid or angry.

figure 1

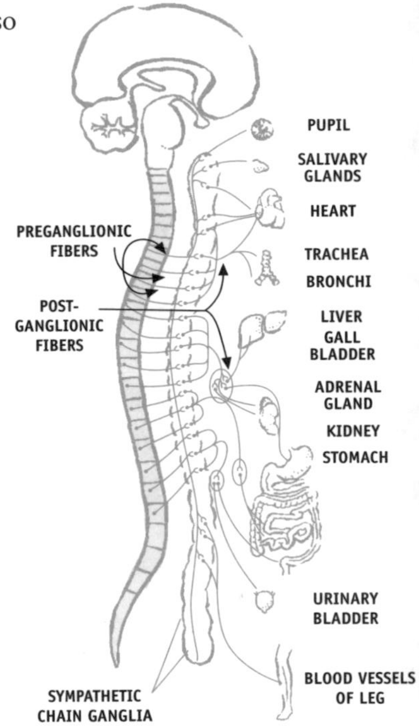

The sympathetic branch is designed instantly to activate the fight-or-flight response. During sympathetic activation the heart rate and heart metabolism increase to prepare the body for action. The blood vessels in the hands, feet, and skin constrict, shunting blood away from the periphery. Presumably this would mean less blood loss in case of injury.

Sympathetic activation also directs the body's resources away from the digestive process. Blood is shunted away from the digestive organs, and peristaltic movement through the intestines is slowed.

THE SYMPATHETIC SYSTEM

In the lungs, sympathetic activation dilates the bronchi and constricts the blood vessels. Breathing rate increases, providing more oxygen for the body. Basal metabolism is increased and more glucose is released into the bloodstream. Metabolism in the muscles is enhanced as well. Sympathetic activation stimulates the adrenal gland to secrete neurotransmitters and hormones to sustain the flight-or-fight response.

There are also sensory and cognitive changes caused by sympathetic activation. The pupil of the eye dilates for improved visual scanning. Mental alertness is increased to help scan the environment.

Sympathetic activation is a well-organized and effective response to danger. Yet if overused, this activation can cause serious health problems, putting direct stress on the heart, disrupting digestion, and depleting energy.

The parasympathetic branch of the autonomic nervous system is organized differently. Neurons emerge from the brain stem and the sacral area of the spinal column. As shown in figure 2, the parasympathetic branch affects many of the same organs as the sympathetic branch, but the parasympathetic system creates a very different internal state,

figure 2

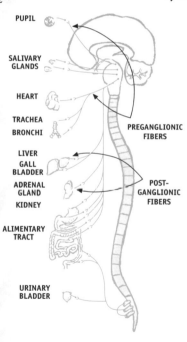

PUPIL

SALIVARY GLANDS

HEART

TRACHEA BRONCHI

LIVER GALL BLADDER

ADRENAL GLAND

KIDNEY

ALIMENTARY TRACT

URINARY BLADDER

PREGANGLIONIC FIBERS

POST-GANGLIONIC FIBERS

THE PARASYMPATHETIC SYSTEM

in which the body is dedicated to nourishment, rest, rebuilding, and healing. In this state, repair and replenishment are priorities.

Parasympathetic activation slows the heart rate and decreases the force of heart contractions. Blood pressure decreases. The bronchi are constricted and blood vessels in the lungs are dilated. Parasympathetic stimulation puts the heart and lungs in a more efficient and restful condition.

Parasympathetic activation supports digestion. Peristaltic movement in the gastrointestinal tract is increased, sphincters in the digestive system are opened, and there is greater blood flow to the GI tract. Parasympathetic activation stimulates the secretion of saliva which helps to start the digestive process in the mouth and stimulates digestive secretions in the stomach. All of this enhances efficient and thorough digestion.

Metabolic rate remains stable so energy supplies are consumed more slowly. The gallbladder, liver, and bladder, stimulated by parasympathetic activation, perform their housekeeping tasks more efficiently. Mentally, parasympathetic activation is associated with a relaxed, satisfied state. Perception is more open. We feel calm.

However, excessive parasympathetic activation can have negative effects. Digestion may proceed too rapidly, leading to frequent bowel movements and poor absorption of food. Asthmatic attacks may be heightened. Mentally and emo-

Parasympathetic stimulation puts the heart and lungs in a more efficient and restful condition.

tionally, we may experience lethargy, weeping, and a sense of hopelessness.

PATTERNS OF AUTONOMIC TENSION

To understand autonomic tension, we need to see the auto nomic nervous system as having two interacting principles of activation and inhibition. We activate our resources to deal with a threat; when it is over, we slow down to rebuild our resources. Activation and inhibition work in balance to make us effective and keep us healthy.

AUTONOMIC ACTIVATION

SYMPATHETIC (ACTIVATION)	PARASYMPATHETIC (INHIBITION)
INCREASES:	**INCREASES:**
Heart rate	Peristalsis
Force of heart contraction	Bronchial constriction
Blood pressure, perspiration	
Sweating, glucose release	
Metabolism, adrenal hormones	
Peripheral vaso constriction	
Mental activity	
Pupil dilation, bronchial dilation	
DECREASES:	**DECREASES:**
Peristalsis	Heart rate
Kidney output	Force of heart contraction
	Blood pressure, perspiration

Autonomic tension occurs when we lose this balance within the ANS. Then we may experience excessive sympathetic activation, excessive parasympathetic activation, or an erratic fluctuation between extreme sympathetic and parasympathetic activations.

The most common type of autonomic tension is excessive sympathetic activation. This is the pattern associated with such destructive stress disorders as heart disease, high blood pressure, insomnia, fatigue, constipation, and digestive problems. People caught in this pattern constantly activate the fight-or-flight response, but seldom return to autonomic balance.

One reason for excessive sympathetic activation is that the ANS seems to be designed to deal with infrequent life-threatening emergencies. The rest of the time, parasympathetic activation takes over. This may have been a good pattern for our hunter-gatherer ancestors who had to respond instantly and intensely when danger was present. The ANS worked perfectly to meet this need.

But the tempo of modern life is very different. Instead of occasional life-threatening dangers, we experience life as a constant attack of minor stressors. The ANS gets turned on during the morning commute and stays turned on all day. Intervals of natural calm and quiet in our environment have mostly vanished. There never seems to be a time for restoring ANS balance. So we experience life in a way that sets off a constant low-grade fight-or-flight response.

Another cause of excessive sympathetic activation is

We experience life in a way that sets off a constant low-grade fight-or-flight response.

rooted in the way the ANS is closely linked with our perception. Any new or unusual stimuli in our environment grabs our attention. If we perceive a threat, we immediately experience an emotional reaction such as fear, which in turn triggers an autonomic response through a part of the brain known as the limbic system.

The limbic system is a brain structure we share with all vertebrates. Birds, snakes, dogs, and cats all have a limbic system which allows them to quickly perceive a threat and instantly activate the flight-or-fight response. Once an emotional reaction is formed in the limbic system, an autonomic response will occur. The more intense the reaction, the greater the ANS response.

This system works well when the organism is dealing with a fairly clear-cut environment. When threats and non-threats are easily distinguished, the limbic system and the ensuing flight-or-fight response work quite well. But for modern humans, the perception of threat and danger is no longer a simple affair. And if we do not appraise events properly, we unnecessarily activate the autonomic nervous system.

Overreacting to events is a frequent cause of excessive sympathetic activation. We get caught in traffic, appraise it as a disaster, and then feel our blood pressure climbing and our stomach churning. Confronted with work deadlines, we label this as an emergency, then notice our heart pounding

For modern humans, the perception of threat and danger is no longer a simple affair.

and our breathing becoming constricted. Countless episodes during the day cause us to overreact and as a result overactivate the ANS.

The second type of autonomic imbalance is excessive parasympathetic activation. This occurs when there is too much inhibition. This pattern can be equally destructive.

This pattern of autonomic tension has been called the "possum response." It is the direct opposite of the fight-or-flight response. Faced with a threat, the opossum does not fight or flee, but shuts down and plays dead. Confronted with overwhelming stress, humans can display a similar response.

There are certain mental patterns associated with this possum response. You are likely to feel despair and hopelessness. You can't see any solution. You feel trapped. When such thoughts and feelings are present, the associated excessive parasympathetic response can cause such symptoms as low energy, restricted breathing, diarrhea, and even sudden death.

The third pattern of autonomic imbalance occurs when we fluctuate between excessive sympathetic and excessive parasympathetic activations. We may feel energized to do battle one moment and feel helpless and trapped the next moment.

This combined autonomic stress is very harmful. It allows for the destructive effects of both kinds of tension

We can learn to utilize specific thought patterns, images, and feeling states to cool down or heat up the ANS.

without the benefits of helpful ANS activation. There is no restoration and housekeeping. There is no effective activation to deal with real problems.

Given the tempo and demands of modern life, it is quite easy to develop autonomic stress. To counter this, we need to learn to rebalance the autonomic nervous system. We can't wait for a quiet existence—we need to create relaxation on the autonomic level.

PRINCIPLES OF AUTONOMIC RELAXATION

The autonomic nervous system is an involuntary system. How can we consciously control it? How can we learn to direct the activity of internal organs?

This all becomes possible if we consider the normal brain pathways that control autonomic responding. Since our thoughts and our emotions normally initiate an ANS response, we can learn to use these to regulate the ANS. We can learn to utilize specific thought patterns, images, and feeling states to cool down or heat up the ANS.

Many of the techniques for autonomic relaxation to be presented in the next chapter involve a combination of mental directives and specific feelings. But there is also a direct physical avenue for achieving autonomic balance.

BREATH: GATEWAY TO
AUTONOMIC REGULATION

Four distinct
dimensions of
breathing affect ANS
activation: inhalation
and exhalation, rate,
thoracic versus
diaphragmatic
breathing, and
finally smoothness.

Breathing is the one physical response that is part of ANS activation and also can be controlled voluntarily. There is even a reciprocal influence: If we start to breathe in a rapid and shallow fashion, this stimulates sympathetic activation. Breathing slowly and evenly stimulates parasympathetic activation. Consequently, we can use our breathing pattern to achieve autonomic balance.

Four distinct dimensions of breathing affect ANS activation: inhalation and exhalation, rate, thoracic versus diaphragmatic breathing, and finally smoothness.

Inhalation is associated with sympathetic activation. When we prepare to fight or flee, we immediately take a deep breath. With each succeeding breath, we inhale vigorously. To provide fuel for fighting and fleeing, we breathe in as much oxygen as possible.

Exhalation, on the other hand, is associated with parasympathetic activation. When danger is past and we feel safe, we often release tension with a long sigh. We continue to exhale strongly in order to cleanse the body of carbon dioxide and restore autonomic balance.

Habitual breathing patterns are linked to autonomic tension. The person locked into a simmering fight-or-flight mode is likely to inhale rapidly, up to twenty to thirty times

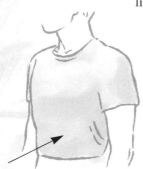

EXHALE

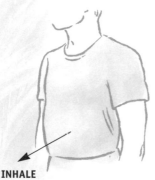

INHALE

Diaphragmatic breathing
is very efficient and
by itself can induce
a calm state.

a minute. The person locked into the possum response is likely to breathe shallowly, with long sighing exhalations, and lives a life without inspiration. In a relaxed state, breathing can slow to a calm and comfortable six to twelve breaths a minute.

The form of the breath varies as well. During a flight-or-fight response, thoracic or chest breathing is typical. This means that the rib cage expands with the inhalation and contracts with the exhalation. This type of breathing can move a great deal of air in and out of the lungs rapidly, providing energy for quick action. But thoracic breathing consumes a great deal of energy and produces a motion in the lungs that sustains and even heightens sympathetic activation.

Diaphragmatic breathing is associated with the relaxation response. In this type of breathing, the abdomen moves out with the inhalation and moves in with the exhalation. The diaphragm, a sheet of muscle under the lungs, moves up with the exhalation, forcing air from the lungs. With inhalation, the diaphragm contracts down, expanding the lungs, allowing air to flow in.

Diaphragmatic breathing is very efficient and by itself can induce a calm state, producing a motion of the lungs that stimulates parasympathetic activation. Diaphragmatic breathing helps you to achieve and sustain a relaxation response.

Smoothness is another dimension to consider. With sympathetic activation, we often gulp for air. The flow of the inhalation is erratic. We may hold our breath at the end of the inhalation. With excessive parasympathetic activation, we may have long irregular exhalations with pauses at the end. These jerks and pauses in the breath indicate autonomic imbalance. To achieve relaxation at the autonomic level, we need to smooth the breath out.

In the next chapter, we will learn breathing techniques, mental procedures, and visualizations to achieve autonomic relaxation.

chapter five

Level II:

autonomic relaxation

techniques

M astering autonomic relaxation is like learning a second language. At first the words may sound strange to us, and our attempts to speak may be halting. But with practice and familiarity, we start to communicate with the subtlest processes in our bodies. As we progress, we become fluent and expressive, until speaking this language becomes second nature.

Like muscular relaxation techniques, autonomic techniques can be grouped into two broad categories: direct and indirect techniques. Let us begin by exploring the direct techniques.

DIRECT METHODS OF AUTONOMIC RELAXATION

Even, Smooth Diaphragmatic Breathing

Diaphragmatic breathing is the most direct technique for reducing autonomic tension. This approach works with the four aspects of the breath that influence autonomic activation: ratio of inhalation to exhalation, type of breath, rate, and smoothness.

The first step is to establish a rhythm of diaphragmatic breathing. In diaphragmatic breathing, when we exhale, the diaphragm relaxes up in a dome shape, compressing the lungs and forcing the air out. When we inhale, the diaphragm contracts downward, pulling the lungs with it.

In the case of diaphragmatic breathing, the abdominal muscles and the diaphragm work together in a synergistic pattern.

This expands the volume of the lungs, creating lower pressure, and air rushes in. This is inspiration.

The lungs are passive participants in respiration. Air is moved in and out of the lungs when muscles expand and shrink the chest cavity. In thoracic breathing, the muscles between the ribs and across the chest expand and contract the chest. In the case of diaphragmatic breathing, the abdominal muscles and the diaphragm work together in a synergistic pattern. When we exhale, we contract the abdominal muscles, pulling them in, the diaphragm relaxes, and air is pushed out. During inhalation we relax the abdominal muscles, the diaphragm contracts down, and air flows into the lungs. Diaphragmatic breathing is illustrated at left.

We don't have direct control over the diaphragm, but we can consciously control the abdominal muscles. The best way to do this is to emphasize the exhalation by pulling the abdominal muscles in, which forces the air out. Then relax your abdominal muscles and a full deep breath will automatically flow in.

In diaphragmatic breathing, the exhalation is the conscious and active part of the breath. If we have a complete exhalation, we can open up to a long, full inhalation. The emphasis on the exhalation

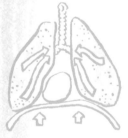

EXHALE

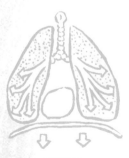

INHALE

may run counter to our typical way of thinking that breathing is improved by taking a deep inhalation. But with diaphragmatic breathing, taking a good breath means starting with a complete exhalation and then just opening up for a full inhalation.

Once you have established diaphragmatic breathing, you can observe the flow of your breathing. You may notice slight hitches and pauses during the cycle of inhalation and exhalation. These irregularities in the breathing pattern are unconscious habits which subtly disturb the flow of the breath and produce stress in the autonomic nervous system. By focusing on your breathing, you can gradually smooth out these hitches and pauses. It is also helpful to make your exhalations and inhalations equal in length. This creates a balance between sympathetic and parasympathetic activation, between excitation and inhibition.

The next step is to slow your breathing. The ancient yogis who devoted considerable study to breathing said that a person's life span is measured not in years but in breaths. The slower the breath, the longer and more vital the life span.

The CD accompanying this book contains a guided practice for diaphragmatic breathing. You should practice even, smooth diaphragmatic breathing for at least ten minutes, twice a day.

The ancient yogis who devoted considerable study to breathing said that a person's life span is measured not in years but in breaths.

Variations: Two-to-One Breathing and Breath Awareness

Two-to-one breathing is a modification of even, smooth diaphragmatic breathing. You simply make the exhalation twice as long as the inhalation. Because the exhalation promotes parasympathetic activation, this breathing slows the system down and induces a relaxation response.

This technique can be used to reduce excessive sympathetic activation, slow the heart rate, decrease blood pressure, and create a calmer, more balanced state. Because two-to-one breathing is so calming, it can also help you fall asleep.

The best way to practice two-to-one breathing is to exhale completely. Then inhale for half of that count. For most people, this means starting with a count of six or eight on the exhalation and three or four on the inhalation. Work within your comfort range. Don't strain. With time and practice, you can gradually lengthen the exhalation and inhalation.

Breath awareness is another technique that can be used after even, smooth diaphragmatic breathing has been

> The best way to practice two-to-one breathing is to exhale completely. Then inhale for half of that count.

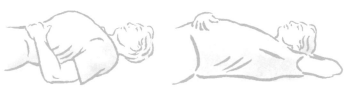

EXHALE   INHALE

mastered. Breath awareness means watching the breath to detect any patterns of imbalance linked to autonomic stress. You might notice that you are holding your breath, inhaling rapidly, breathing from your chest, or exhaling with a long sigh. When you notice these signs of tension, you can guide your breathing back to even, smooth diaphragmatic breathing. This will reduce any autonomic tension that has begun to accumulate.

There are two ways to practice breath awareness. The first is to anchor a moment of breath awareness to a specific activity. For instance, each time you get in the car, you might direct your awareness to your breath. Or each time you end a telephone call and hang up the phone, you could check your breathing pattern to see if patterns of tension are present. Such frequent associations provide regular opportunities to practice breath awareness.

The second method of breath awareness involves dedicating a part of your mind to continually monitor and be aware of your breathing. This takes more practice. As you are walking, working, reading, or listening, part of your mind is watching your breathing for signs of tension. When tension arises, you spontaneously smooth it out and prevent escalation.

Autogenic Relaxation
Autogenic training is another direct method for achieving

Breath awareness means watching the breath to detect any patterns of imbalance linked to autonomic stress.

relaxation at the autonomic level. The term "autogenic" refers to a self-generated state of relaxation in which autonomic balance is restored and the recuperative powers of the body are activated.

Autogenic training originated with the work of Dr. Oskar Vogt in Berlin, Germany, in the 1890s. Experimenting with hypnosis, Vogt observed that subjects who learned to enter a self-induced hypnotic state consistently reported feelings of heaviness and warmth during the session and afterward felt rested and restored. When subjects created this state on a daily basis, they reported decreased fatigue and tension, fewer headaches, and increased energy.

In follow-up work during the early 1900s, Dr. Johannes Schultz was looking for a therapeutic method that utilized the benefits of hypnosis but avoided the passivity of the patient and the dependence on a therapist. Noting that during the initial stages of hypnosis, patients consistently reported their limbs felt relaxed and heavy and their body felt agreeably warm, he instructed subjects to create these sensations. When he obtained good results, he added directives to relax the rhythm of the heart and to smooth out respiration. To mimic the effects of warm baths and cool compresses, he told his trainees to think of warmth in the abdominal region and coolness in the forehead. These six specific physiological effects became the foundation

The term "autogenic" refers to a self-generated state of relaxation in which autonomic balance is restored and the recuperative powers of the body are activated.

of autogenic training. They were formulated into specific phrases that subjects repeated internally to create the relaxing effects.

Schultz also discovered that autogenic relaxation was best achieved through passive concentration. There should be rapt attention, he wrote, but not a feeling of struggle. There should be a sense of letting things happen, encouraging them but not forcing them to happen.

Passive concentration is achieved by following systematic steps. First, select a quiet environment and wear loose, comfortable clothes. Second, as you silently repeat the autogenic phrases, make mental contact with the body and generate a flow of visual, tactile, and auditory images to support the effect of the phrase. For example, while repeating, "My heartbeat is calm and regular," you might hear the steady heartbeat, visualize it, and feel it in your chest. The images should be comfortable, pleasant, and effective for you.

During the practice of autogenic relaxation, your attention may drift or you may get so relaxed that you move into a sleep state. Any time you notice that you have lost your focus, start over with the phrase you were using.

To practice autogenic relaxation, follow the guided instructions on the CD that comes with this book. Or assume the Shavasana relaxation pose, utilize passive concentration, and repeat each of the following autogenic phrases three times.

> During the practice of autogenic relaxation, your attention may drift or you may get so relaxed that you move into a sleep state.

My right arm is heavy.
My left arm is heavy.
Both arms are heavy.
My right leg is heavy.
My left leg is heavy.
Both legs are heavy.
My right arm is warm.
My left arm is warm.
Both arms are warm.
My right leg is warm.
My left leg is warm.
Both legs are warm.
My arms and legs are heavy and warm.
My heartbeat is calm and regular.
It breathes me.
My solar plexus is warm.
My forehead is cool.

Autogenic relaxation can help to relieve a wide variety of disorders associated with ANS tension, including digestive problems, cardiovascular disease, hypertension, asthma, insomnia, headaches, and back pain. With regular practice, autogenic relaxation increases energy, vitality, and overall health.

Rotation of Consciousness

In the chapter on muscular relaxation, a subtle technique known as Rotation of Consciousness was introduced. This approach involved guiding awareness to different muscle groups throughout the body. The underlying idea was that muscular tension is maintained by a lack of awareness.

There is also a Rotation of Consciousness technique for the autonomic level, involving moving awareness through a number of centers in the body linked to autonomic functioning. These include some of the points we learned about in autogenic relaxation chapter, such as the forehead, throat, heart, solar plexus, and lower abdomen. But there are also a number of more subtle autonomic centers related to the energy pathways or meridians of acupuncture. In yoga, these energy channels are called *nadis*. Their main junctions or intersections are called *chakras*, meaning "wheels of energy."

This Rotation of Consciousness exercise is designed to guide awareness along the major autonomic centers and energy pathways. Known as the sixty-one points, this procedure creates

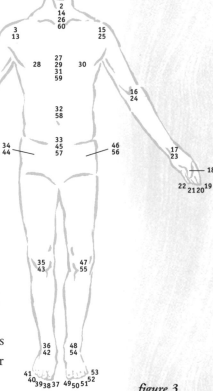

figure 3

**This method
entails making
and sustaining
mental contact
with each point.**

profound relaxation at the autonomic level. The sixty-one points are illustrated in figure 3.

This method entails making and sustaining mental contact with each point. Sometimes people will have difficulty making contact with a certain part of their body. This may mean that the energy flow to that area is weaker, indicating autonomic tension and blocked energy flow. When you reestablish contact with that part of the body, tension is reduced and energy flow is improved.

Most people have so much autonomic tension that they will benefit from working with breathing and autogenic techniques. But once these foundation techniques are mastered and some degree of balance has been restored to the ANS, Rotation of Consciousness can be used to achieve an even deeper and more profound relaxation. Bringing awareness to the autonomic nervous system and the related energy pathways is also a very integrating experience.

To practice the sixty-one points technique, you can memorize the points from figure 3 and then guide your awareness through the sequence of points, maintaining awareness at each point for three to five seconds. Or you can tape-record the guided practice below.

After you go through the sixty-one points the first time, repeat the procedure with deeper awareness. Remember to maintain a feeling of non-effort and non-striving.

the
practice

- Stretch out on your back and assume the Shavasana pose. Notice the spots where your body is making contact with the floor and just let go at each of those spots. Establish even, smooth diaphragmatic breathing.

- Bring your awareness to the forehead. Make mental contact with the forehead. Think of the number 1. Hold your awareness at your forehead for five seconds. Move your awareness to the throat and think 2. Bring your awareness to your right shoulder and think 3. Guide your awareness to the right elbow and think 4. Make mental contact with the right wrist and think 5. Now make mental contact with each finger. Start by guiding your attention to the right thumb, number 6, the right index finger, number 7; the right middle finger is number 8, the right ring finger, number 9, and the right little finger, number 10.

- Bring your awareness back to the right wrist, number 11, to the right elbow, number 12, to the right shoulder, number 13, and back to the throat, number 14. Make mental contact with your left shoulder, number 15, then your left elbow, number 16, and your left wrist, number 17. Guide your awareness to each finger of the left hand. Start with the left thumb, number 18, left index finger, number 19, left middle finger, number 20, left ring finger, number 21, and left little finger, number 22.

- Move your awareness to the left wrist, number 23, to the left elbow, number 24, to the left shoulder, number 25 and back to the throat, number 26. Bring your awareness to the heart center, number 27. Guide your attention to the right nipple, number 28, back to the heart center, number 29, to the left nipple, number 30, and back to the heart center for 31.

- Now bring your awareness to the navel center, number 32, and then to the pelvic center, number 33. Move your awareness to the right hip, number 34, to the right knee, 35, and to the right ankle, 36. Bring your attention to the right big toe, 37, the second toe, 38, the middle toe, 39, the fourth toe, 40, and the little toe, 41. Move your awareness back to the right ankle, 42, to the right knee, 43, the right hip, 44, and back to the pelvic center, 45.

- Next, bring your attention to the left hip, 46, the left knee, 47, and the left ankle, 48. Guide your awareness to the left big toe, 49, the second toe, 50, the middle toe, 51, the fourth toe, 52, and the little toe, 53. Bring your awareness back to the left ankle, 54, the left knee, 55, and the left hip, 56.

- Direct your awareness to the pelvic center, 57, the navel center, 58, the heart center, 59, the throat center, 60, and the forehead center, 61.

- Now go through all sixty-one points a second time. Stay

with each point a little longer. Deepen the focus at each point.

• When you have finished with the second sixty-one points, bring your awareness back to your breathing. Take several deeper breaths. Let a sense of activity return to your hands and feet. Gently wiggle your fingers and toes. Bring your arms up over your head and take a long, lazy stretch. Open your eyes and notice the world around you. Also notice the inner feelings and sensations of relaxation, autonomic balance, and integration. When you are ready, open your eyes and gently move back into the activities of the day, keeping an awareness of autonomic balance.

Bring your arms up over your head and take a long, lazy stretch. Open your eyes and notice the world around you.

INDIRECT METHODS OF AUTONOMIC RELAXATION

Exercise

Exercise is as helpful for reducing autonomic tension as it is for easing muscular tension. During the course of a stressful day, autonomic tension builds; heart rate climbs, blood pressure rises, and breathing becomes choppy and constricted. Vigorous or aerobic exercise releases this tension. Running, swimming, biking, or briskly walking starts by

Vigorous exercise is particularly helpful for loosening up and normalizing the breathing.

increasing heart rate and blood pressure. But after the exercise, heart rate and blood pressure drop to a normal level and we feel a sense of release and calm.

Vigorous exercise is particularly helpful for loosening up and normalizing the breathing. When we run or bike we are forced to take fuller and deeper breaths. After exercise, breathing is smoother, deeper, and slower.

Exercise also helps to stir us out of a helpless "possum" mentality. When we exercise vigorously we overcome lethargy and passivity. Exercise is energizing. It gives us a sense of accomplishment and encourages optimism.

The type of aerobic exercise performed is a matter of individual preference. Three to four sessions of exercise a week is very beneficial. The exercise should be demanding enough to raise the heart rate for about twenty minutes.

When exercising, try to avoid an attitude of struggle. Keep an easy, comfortable attitude. Work within your comfortable capacity. Try to maximize the beneficial effect on breathing by coordinating your breathing with the exercise and evening out inhalation and exhalation.

Visualization

Visualization is another effective indirect method for achieving autonomic relaxation, working with the emotional and mental centers that control the autonomic nervous system. When we vividly picture a scene, we occupy the mind with a positive image. This crowds out all the stressful thoughts that normally would be creating tension in the ANS. When the content of the visualization is pleasing, it creates a tranquil or pleasant emotional state which reduces sympathetic responding and restores autonomic balance.

The key elements of effective visualization are vivid imagery and positive, pleasing, or inspiring content. When all the senses are employed and the mind is completely absorbed in a beautiful scene, feelings of joy and tranquility emerge.

One of the most effective visualizations is "The Favorite Place," where you picture a favorite place in nature. It might be a beach, a forest, or a mountain you have known, a composite of places you have known, or a place you create in your imagination. The important thing is to utilize all the senses to visualize that place.

the
practice

• Select a quiet, comfortable room with a soft carpet. Stretch out on your back and assume the Shavasana relaxation pose. Take several deep breaths, then establish even, smooth diaphragmatic breathing. Release any

One of the most effective visualizations is "The Favorite Place," where you picture a favorite place in nature.

unnecessary tension from the arms and legs. Relax your face muscles.

- In your mind, begin to picture your favorite place, a natural setting known to you. Experience a very specific aspect of that place with one of your senses, such as the sense of touch. For example, if it is the beach, you might start by feeling the texture of the sand under your feet. Notice how smooth it is and how deep your feet sink into the sand. Then vividly feel another aspect, such as the temperature of the sand.

- As these feeling experiences become established, shift to another sense. Vividly hear a specific sound. It might be the sound of the wind, the flow or lapping of water, the rustling of leaves or the song of a bird. Then let yourself hear another sound.

- As those experiences are established, move your attention to the visual channel and see some specific aspect of the setting. It might be a color, a shape, or a vista. See it clearly. Then see another specific aspect of your setting.

- Perhaps you can even notice some specific fragrance or smell that is part of your setting. Possibly you can notice the smell of the ocean or of pine needles. Maybe the air even has a unique taste.

- Allow yourself to become immersed in this natural setting. Open yourself up to feelings of peace and well-being

In your mind, begin to picture your favorite place, a natural setting known to you. Experience a very specific aspect of that place with one of your senses, such as the sense of touch.

that emerge. Feel yourself opening to the natural rhythms of this setting.

- Go back through the senses one at a time. Feel another specific aspect of the setting. Hear another sound. See another color or shape. Notice another smell or taste. Notice new things in your favorite place. Deepen the experience of your favorite place. Partake of the inherent tranquility and balance of the setting. You can even let your imagination create new things there.

- When you are ready, bring your awareness back to your breathing. Let your breathing become a little more active. Bring your awareness to your hands and feet. Gently wiggle your fingers and toes. Open your eyes. Reach your hands up over your head and take a nice long stretch. Whenever you are ready, come back up to a seated position. Resume the activities of the day. Take the feeling of autonomic balance and deep inner relaxation with you.

Reach your hands up over your head and take a nice long stretch...Take the feeling of autonomic balance and deep inner relaxation with you.

After six months of regular autonomic relaxation, you will be sleeping better and stress symptoms such as digestive problems, anxiety, high blood pressure, and headaches will have lessened or disappeared.

GUIDELINES FOR PRACTICE

Autonomic relaxation should be practiced on a daily basis over a number of months. It takes time to reprogram the autonomic nervous system from a state of constant tension to a state of balance and relaxation. As you master the techniques of autonomic relaxation, several important changes will occur. First of all, your ANS will gradually shift to a more balanced state. Secondly, you will develop a "training effect," i.e., you will be able to achieve autonomic relaxation more quickly. To begin with, it might take twenty minutes to achieve a mild degree of autonomic relaxation. But after six months you will be able to achieve deep autonomic relaxation in five to ten minutes.

After six months of regular autonomic relaxation, you will be sleeping better and stress symptoms such as digestive problems, anxiety, high blood pressure, and headaches will have lessened or disappeared. Mental clarity and emotional balance will improve. The stage will be set to learn relaxation techniques for the emotional, mental, and spiritual levels.

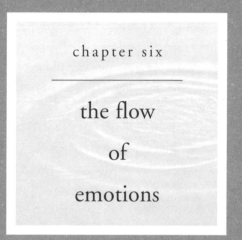

chapter six

_____

the flow

of

emotions

E motions play a central role in the way we experience each moment of life. They influence our thoughts, shape our behavior, and trigger reactions throughout our body. Emotions can energize and inspire us to accomplish amazing feats. Yet emotions can weaken us to the point where it is a struggle to get through the day.

Negative emotions have specific physical effects. Anxiety makes our stomach churn. Anger raises our blood pressure. Worry gives us a headache. Fear makes us feel cold inside. Despair drains our energy.

Emotions can also have positive physical effects. A relaxed person emanates peace and tranquility. A smile immediately softens muscular tension in the face and throughout the body. And love brings energy and enthusiasm.

Because emotions play such a pivotal role in our lives, learning to manage them is a key element in creating total relaxation. We need to understand the nature of emotions, the causes of emotional tension, and the principles of emotional relaxation. Then we will be ready to learn the methods of emotional relaxation.

EMOTIONS DEFINED

The word "emotion" is derived from the Latin verb *exmovere,* "to move away." "Emotion" is defined as a state of

Because emotions play such a pivotal role in our lives, learning to manage them is a key element in creating total relaxation.

feeling combined with a strong physical response that prepares the body for immediate, vigorous action.

Emotions have inherent survival and protective value. When we sense danger, fear can mobilize us to run and escape. When we experience anger, we tighten up our muscles and are ready to fight. Emotions also give us energy us to create and achieve. When we are infused with enthusiasm, we can accomplish incredible feats and overcome obstacles. Feelings of love for a child give us the energy and stamina to protect that child.

There are actually a small number of basic emotions. These include anger, sadness, fear, disgust, shame, surprise, happiness, peacefulness, and love. These basic emotions are so central to human experience that some of them— anger, fear, sadness, and happiness—produce characteristic facial expressions recognized by people all over the world. A Native American Eskimo, an Australian Aborigine, and a European city dweller all know what an angry face looks like.

These basic emotions are more like names for a family of related feelings. For example, anger can vary from mild irritation to absolute fury. Fear spans the continuum from edginess to absolute terror. Happiness may range from pleased to ecstatic.

Emotions can therefore combine to create complex states of feeling. Depression often combines sadness, fear, disgust, and anger. For different people, depression may be a different blend of these core feelings. Depression may even take different forms for the same person.

If you observe your emotions arise, you may notice two stages. The first is an immediate feeling reaction linked to instantaneous physiological changes. The second stage is more mental in nature and involves thinking about the event and noting the feelings occurring.

Imagine you are walking down a street in an unfamiliar neighborhood at night. Suddenly you hear footsteps approaching behind you. Your immediate and instinctive emotional reaction is fear. Instantly your heart starts racing, your breath speeds up, and your muscles tense in readiness to flee.

Following this strong initial reaction, a number of secondary reactions occur. You have awareness of your fear. You may try to control your fear by thinking. "Stay calm." "Don't look afraid." "Keep walking in a steady, confident manner." Or you might have thoughts that intensify the fear. "I'm going to be mugged." "I'm caught and I can't help myself."

These two phases of emotional reaction reflect different brain pathways. The first reaction is controlled by more primitive brain structures that we have in common with other animals. Dogs and wolves have this type of instant emotional reaction. When threatened, they immediately growl and snarl, ready to fight or flee. There is no thinking involved in this reaction. It is immediate.

The first stage is an immediate feeling reaction linked to instantaneous physiological changes. The second stage is more mental in nature and involves thinking about the event and noting the feelings occurring.

The second phase of the emotional reaction is uniquely human and draws on neural pathways in the higher cortical regions of the brain. It is these areas that allow us to be conscious of our feelings and to think about the event that triggered the emotional reaction. During this second phase, our thoughts can operate to decrease the emotional reaction or to heighten and sustain the emotional response.

This second phase of the emotional response gives us the capacity to regulate and control our emotions. By thinking things over, we can work through emotional turbulence.

But there are also disadvantages with this cognitive control system. We can choose to suppress even the strongest emotions. Or we can continue to upset ourselves about events that have long since ceased to be any type of threat. We can even imagine threats that aren't there. It is this aspect of the cognitive control system that often leads to emotional tension.

EMOTIONAL TENSION

Strong emotions are designed to be of short duration. Emotional tension occurs when negative emotions persist, whether overt or suppressed. This persistence is a uniquely human problem. In other animals, negative

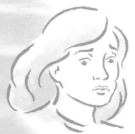

STAGE 1
Immediate person feels fear

STAGE 2
Delayed person is worried, concerned, and afraid

emotions are expressed strongly and completely, but then quickly fade away.

When my dog chases another dog away, she is in a full-fledged fighting mode. The hair on her back stands up, her lips are curled back, her fangs are showing. Her heart is racing and her body is fully mobilized to fight. But as soon as the other dog leaves, she begins to relax. And ten minutes later she can be curled up at my feet, drowsing peacefully. I am sure she is not fuming about the bad manners of the other dog. She is not troubled by thoughts that the other dog might come back next week. Nor is she worrying about how she handled the situation.

All of these concerns are, however, typical of humans. We have the ability to make negative emotions persist. When we have an argument with the boss, or make some dumb mistake, we can replay the event in our minds and feel upset for hours, days, weeks, and even years. At any time in the future we can rerun the incident and reignite our anger and frustration.

We can also create further emotional turbulence by conjuring up complex and frightening scenarios of a future disaster, by picturing in our mind how we might get fired, go bankrupt, lose our house, suffer rejection from family and friends, and die in abject poverty. All these thought patterns create and sustain strong negative emotions.

Negative emotions are often self-perpetuating. When

We can also create further emotional turbulence by conjuring up complex and frightening scenarios of a future disaster.

we feel sad, we selectively notice things that make us even sadder and we ignore the things that could make us happy. When we are filled with anger, we tend to see and hear those things which irritate us and make us even more angry.

Emotional tension creates excessive activation and tension at the muscular and autonomic levels. Changes may also occur at a biochemical level. Persistent feelings of discouragement and sadness may deplete the brain of neurotransmitters that normally elevate mood. As a result, it may become progressively harder to experience happiness. When this happens, you can become locked in a state of emotional tension.

TRIGGERS FOR NEGATIVE EMOTIONS

There are many events that trigger negative emotions and lead to emotional tension. The most common cause is when something happens contrary to our wants and preferences. It might be something that somebody else does or says that evokes a negative emotion. Or we may do or say something we don't like. Negative emotions can also be triggered by major life events such as illness, financial problems, relationship difficulties, job changes, or the death of a family member.

A strong emotional response to upsetting events and life stressors is natural. But it is our tendency to sustain and exacerbate negative emotions that turns healthy emotional responses into emotional tension. The ways we think about, talk to ourselves about, or visualize the event are the brain activities that sustain emotional tension.

Suggestions are another source of emotional tension. We are all influenced by the same power of suggestion hypnotists use to direct people to behave unusually or to feel sensations of heat or cold. Our emotions are influenced by the negative and positive suggestions of others. This attachment to the suggestions of others puts us on an emotional roller coaster.

Basic instincts are another source of emotions. The famous psychiatrist/neurologist Sigmund Freud believed the instinct for sexual pleasure was the basic driving force of our emotional life.

Practitioners of yoga believe that there are actually four basic urges that drive human behavior: self-preservation, food, sex, and sleep. Emotions arise when we think about these needs, when we satisfy these urges, or when our attempts to satisfy these urges are frustrated.

As an example, consider how our emotions are constantly affected by our need for food. We worry about when to eat, what to eat, and how much to eat. We want to satisfy the need for food. We want to enjoy our food. But all too often we experience guilt, anxiety, and disappointment about our food.

> Practitioners of yoga believe that there are actually four basic urges that drive human behavior: self-preservation, food, sex, and sleep.

If we study our feelings over the course of the day, we can see that the other three basic urges—self-preservation, sex, and sleep—create similar patterns of emotions. Our instinct for self-preservation ignites strong emotional responses if we encounter any type of physical danger or threat. On a more subtle level, self-preservation is threatened when people criticize or reject us.

The need for sleep also influences our emotions. When we enjoy a good night's sleep we feel rested and happy. But if our sleep is restless or interrupted, we will feel irritable and short-tempered. If we are deprived of our sleep for any length of time, we can become mentally unstable. When we are unable to satisfy any of these urges, we experience emotional tension.

Another source of negative emotions is early childhood trauma. Children who live through a frightening event may live with deep feelings of fear and develop a core belief that the world is a dangerous and scary place. Children who are humiliated or abused may harbor rage deep in their psyche. Children who experience traumatic loss may feel underlying sadness and hopelessness throughout their life.

THE EFFECTS OF EMOTIONAL TENSION

Chronic negative emotions affect us in many ways. Negative emotions are directly and immediately linked to muscular and autonomic activation. Consequently, emotional tension can cause many physical symptoms, including headaches, back pain, digestive problems, hypertension, and heart disease. Emotional tension decreases the vitality of our immune system and depletes our energy reserves.

Emotional tension also influences our perception. When we have persistent fear, we begin to selectively look for danger. With underlying anxiety, we are constantly scanning the environment for things that could go wrong. With constant sadness and hopelessness, we see limitations and barriers everywhere. The glass is always half empty. And if we have a pattern of enduring anger, we are quick to notice things that irritate and provoke us.

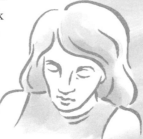

Emotional tension decreases the vitality of our immune system and depletes our energy reserves.

Emotional tension disrupts our basic life rhythms. When we are angry, anxious, or depressed, we either can't fall asleep or we sleep too much. And when we are upset, we either lose our appetite completely or continually engage in nervous eating. When our sleeping and eating are disrupted, we feel even worse physically and emotionally. We are less likely to exercise or undertake any positive actions that would make us feel better.

Emotional tension also restricts our natural emotional spontaneity. When we are gripped by persistent anger or anxiety, it is very difficult to respond to the simple joys

When we are gripped by persistent anger or anxiety, it is very difficult to respond to the simple joys around us.

around us. We become blind to the inspiring beauty of nature. We are unable to accept kindness and love from others. Ironically, persistent emotional tension even prevents us from getting angry or sad in a spontaneous and natural manner.

This tension also blocks our natural tendency toward self-development. If we are gripped by persistent negative emotions, our life takes on a reactive, driven quality. The little boy with buried rage organizes his life around never again being humiliated. The little girl filled with anxiety is driven to control everything and everybody in her life. When we build our lives around reacting to emotional tension, it is difficult to enter on a path of growth where we are inspired toward some ideal or goal.

Emotional tension affects our relationships. In the closeness of an intimate relationship, it is impossible to hide or cover up our underlying emotional tension. Inevitably, we project our emotional issues into the relationship. If we bring fear into the relationship, we soon begin to doubt our partner. If we bring anger into the relationship, it won't be long before we feel anger toward our partner. In both instances we simply end up reinforcing our patterns of emotional tension.

THE NATURE OF EMOTIONAL RELAXATION

Simply put, emotional relaxation means letting go of negative feelings. Many people believe that this is impossible. They believe that their negative emotions have a firm grip on them. They identify fully with the reality of being sad, discouraged, or angry. With emotional relaxation, we learn to break free from the grasp of anxiety, fear, and sadness.

Then negative emotions begin to function the way they should. Arising in response to an event, they provide us with the energy to respond in a protective or assertive manner and then return to a more balanced state.

Emotional relaxation is more than just decreasing negative emotions. When we release negative emotions, positive emotions move to the foreground of our experience. A secondary goal of emotional relaxation is to encourage and enhance a wide spectrum of positive emotions.

These positive emotions fall into several broad categories. The first category contains such terms as contentment, serenity, peacefulness, tranquility, and calmness. Feelings of quietude and peace, experienced all too infrequently, can arise naturally when we let go of negative emotions.

Another category of positive emotions deals with a more active sense of enjoyment and includes pleasure, joy,

> With emotional relaxation, we learn to break free from the grasp of anxiety, fear, and sadness.

Feelings of
quietude and
peace, experienced
all too infrequently,
can arise naturally
when we let go of
negative emotions.

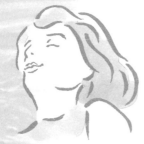

delight, bliss, rapture, and ecstasy. In a state of emotional relaxation, we are more open to these naturally occurring emotions. There is no need to be thrill seekers; we are able to experience these emotions through time spent with family or friends, listening to music, reading, taking a walk, or completing a job or project.

A third category of positive emotions deals with expressions of love. This category includes friendliness, acceptance, affinity, devotion, and adoration. These feelings can be directed toward a person, an ideal, a creative process, or a specific goal in life. These feelings of love fulfill, inspire, and energize us.

Positive emotions have a beneficial effect on our body. Serenity brings physical peacefulness and rest. Enjoyment is energizing, and love seems to actually change our brain chemistry, releasing neurotransmitters that make us feel good.

Emotional relaxation also changes the way we experience time. Emotional tension locks us into the past and the future. We worry about what has happened. We fret about what might happen. Consequently, we miss most of what is happening in the present. We are able to experience the present only through the filters created by past experience and future worries.

But with emotional relaxation all of this changes. When we let go of negative emotions, our awareness naturally moves into the present. We become more open and aware of what is happening. We truly see, hear, and touch the world around us. We perceive the choices and opportunities available in the present.

When we reduce emotional tension, we are able to live life more fully, to work creatively, and to love in a natural and healthy manner. We become more spontaneous, more balanced, and more in charge of our life.

chapter seven

Level III:
emotional relaxation

techniques

B ecause thoughts play a crucial role in maintaining and heightening negative emotions, there are a number of emotional relaxation techniques that work with thoughts. These are the *cognitive approaches.*

Because emotions create physiological activation, there are a number of physical techniques for emotional relaxation. And, because emotions arise from four basic instinctual needs or urges, we need to understand and work with these urges in order to achieve emotional balance.

COGNITIVE APPROACHES TO EMOTIONAL RELAXATION

Revising Self-Talks

Some of the most persistent negative emotions are inextricably linked to patterns of thinking. Consider a person who is depressed. He thinks that his life is heading downhill and will never improve. He sees himself as ineffectual and believes he can never change. These thoughts occur in his mind as self-talks. A depressed person repeats these *self-talks* over and over.

Distinct patterns of self-talks create distinct patterns of emotional tension. Anxious people tell themselves that everything will go wrong, that the consequences of a mistake will be ruinous, and that everyone is thinking the worst of them. Angry people tell themselves they're not going to let anyone get the best of them, that they have to always have the last word, and that they must get even for any insult.

Revising self-talks is an important method for achieving emotional relaxation. We can start by learning to listen to and notice the content of our self-talks. When we are caught up in persistent anger or anxiety, we should notice what we are telling ourselves. Then we can replace our tension-producing self-talks with thoughts that reduce negative emotions and cultivate a positive state.

Self-talks that produce negative emotions can be grouped into six categories: *demands, denial, overreacting, always-never thinking, all-or-nothing thinking,* and *mind reading.* Let's examine each category of harmful self-talk and explore ways to revise them.

Demands

The first category consists of the rigid and at times unrealistic demands that we make of others, of ourselves, and of life in general. In our internal language these demands are typically couched in words such as "should," "must be," and "have to." Our spouse *should* be understanding, patient, and loving. We feel that our colleagues *must* be fair and show us respect. We expect that traffic *should* run smoothly, that our car *should* work correctly after we have had it repaired, that our efforts *should* be recognized and rewarded.

When our demands aren't met, we get upset. We get angry at others, at ourselves, or at life in general. We tend to repeat our demands over and over, and our anger grows, eventually turning into chronic emotional tension.

We often try to justify our demands, referring to "what is right" and "what I would do," and holding other people to our own standards. Most of the time, our demands are nothing more than our desires.

Once we realize that the core of any demand is a desire or want, we can begin to change it. We can restate our demands in a more reasonable manner: "I would *like* my spouse to be understanding, patient, and loving. "I would *prefer* to have respect and fair treatment from my colleagues." "I *like* it when traffic runs smoothly and my car works."

At first glance, these changes in our inner language may seem slight and inconsequential, a matter of semantics. But, in fact, these changes create certain shifts. When we think of our desires in terms of wants and preferences rather than rigid demands, we create more flexibility in our emotional response and often in the responses of others. We aren't as attached to the outcome. We recognize that we don't get everything we want.

If we examine our desires, we may find that some of them aren't really that important, but are internalized

Rephrasing expectations from the rigid language of "shoulds" and "musts" to preferences and wants is the first step in revising our self-talks.

expectations and suggestions from family and society. On the other hand, if we do want something, stating it clearly as a want can transform it into an ideal that inspires us and gives us feelings of hope, enthusiasm, and energy.

Rephrasing expectations from the rigid language of "shoulds" and "musts" to preferences and wants is the first step in revising our self-talks.

Denial

The second category of stress-producing self-talks is denial. In this case, we use our inner language to deny the reality of an event. When someone betrays our trust, we might think, "I just can't believe this happened" or "I can't believe he did that." A second type of denial involves lack of insight into an event. In this case our self-talks might be "How could anybody do that?" or "I just don't understand." When we continually repeat these self-talks, we feel increasingly perplexed, anxious, and upset.

We can deal with the first type of denial by doing a reality check, acknowledge that the event did indeed happen, and then move on. For the second type of denial, we can realize that events usually have multiple causes. We just need time, effort, and the right perspective to see the causes of someone else's or our own behavior. We can also understand and accept that at times people act impulsively and unpredictably.

Overreacting

When we repeat to ourselves that an event is horrible and awful and that we can't stand it, we are overreacting. The more we repeat these extreme evaluations, the more upset we get. Even a few moments of overreacting will lead to a full-blown fight-or-flight response.

When we fall into the pattern of overreacting, it no longer matters what the event is. We could be upset about something as minor as misplacing car keys or getting a parking ticket. But when we react to this event with defeating self-talks, we will create strong negative emotions. Then when we are confronted with a major life event such as loss of a job, the end of a relationship, or a death in the family, our habitual overreacting will prevent us from accepting and adjusting to this trauma.

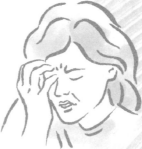

There are several important insights that will help us to revise the self-talks of overreacting. To begin with, we can understand that nothing is inherently horrible or terrible. It is our interpretation of an event that makes it horrible or awful.

We can also consider how our reactions to events change over time. What seemed horrible five years ago can now be viewed with equanimity. With the passage of time, we gain a different perspective on events. One technique to help us gain this perspective is called the Five Method.

Nothing is inherently horrible or terrible. It is our interpretation of an event that makes it horrible or awful.

When confronting an apparent crisis, ask yourself how you will feel about it in five years. And if that seems OK, then ask yourself how you will feel in five months. When that feels OK, pose the question for five weeks, five days, five hours, and even five minutes.

With the passage of time, we can discover surprising aspects to apparently grim events. Failing out of school, losing a job, or breaking off a relationship may have seemed terrible when it happened. But when we view the event now, we may discern a positive side. Over the course of a lifetime, these seemingly horrible events were way stations that ultimately led us to a better school, a more satisfying job, or a better relationship.

The Five Method provides us with a powerful technique for reframing negative events. The trick is to not wait five years to cope with an event, but to immediately find opportunities in seemingly negative events. When a door is closed, we can look for the window that has opened.

Always-Never Thinking
Always-never self-talks involve projecting our overreactions into the future. We tell ourselves we will always perform poorly, always make a mess out of things, and always make poor choices. We think that we will always feel sad, abandoned, lonely, and unloved. We tell ourselves we will never succeed, never reach our potential, never do things right.

These always-never self-talks have an extremely negative effect on our emotions and physical well-being. They present a contradictory message to the nervous system and muscles. On one hand, we are telling ourselves that something is very wrong, which leads to activation. Yet at the same time, we are telling ourselves nothing can be done, which leads to inhibition. It is like pressing the gas pedal and the brakes at the same time.

We can revise these self-talks by considering the nature of emotions. Negative feelings will fade away unless they are reinforced by counter-productive self-talks. Consequently, we can tell ourselves these feelings will pass, that we will recover, we will bounce back.

Just as emotions fade and change, so do circumstances. What falls in the category of "never" today might easily be possible next week. What seems a chronic condition now could change in the future. We can be patient and look for the right time, when things are ready to change. For example, many people believed the Berlin Wall would stand for a long time to come, yet when the time was right, it fell with surprising speed.

We can also search for those first steps, the beginning actions that will help rid us of always-never thinking. When we act to improve things, no matter how small or symbolic the act, we provide evidence to support our more optimistic self-talks.

What falls in the category of "never" today might easily be possible next week.

With all-or-nothing thinking, we become caught up in the fallacy that one behavior describes the complete person and that one event portrays the complete situation.

All-or-Nothing Thinking

With all-or-nothing thinking, we make absolute evaluations of ourselves and others. If we commit a social error, we conclude that we are totally without social skills. If we make a blunder at work, we tell ourselves we are totally incompetent. If another person lies to us or manipulates us in some way, we think he or she is inconsiderate and totally rotten.

With all-or-nothing thinking, we become caught up in the fallacy that one behavior describes the complete person and that one event portrays the complete situation. When we react to life this way, we significantly increase our anger, frustration, and sadness. When we are enmeshed in all-or-nothing thinking, we can't see solutions, options, and possibilities. We are unable to recognize the positive aspects of ourselves or others.

To revise all-or-nothing self-talks, we need to gain a broader perspective and accept the mistake. Then we can forgive ourselves, learn what we can from it, and make a commitment to handle things differently in the future. We can also remind ourselves of our better side, of our skills and our friendships.

Mind Reading

Mind reading occurs when we believe that our tension, our anxieties, our physical flaws, and our apparel defects are glaringly visible to others. If we are giving a talk in front of a large audience, we are convinced everyone can hear the slight tremor in our voice, see the shakiness of our hand, and sense our nervous perspiration.

Once these self-talks about the thoughts of others start racing through our mind, we create a cycle of making ourselves more anxious and possibly drawing more attention to our problems. We become even more self-conscious and tense and are more likely to make mistakes. We find ourselves avoiding people, avoiding situations, and projecting a negative image.

These mind-reading self-talks can be revised by realizing that others rarely perceive our inner reactions. You may be at the podium and notice your heart rate pounding and your hands sweating. But a member of the audience, even if he or she notices your nervousness, gives it only passing attention or reacts sympathetically.

It is not healthy or logical to become worried about the evaluations of other. Certainly we can listen, take in feedback, and learn from it. But we want to break out of the trap of excessive mind reading. After

CATEGORY	NEGATIVE SELF TALK	POSITIVE SELF TALK
Demands	I, he, you should, must	I would like, prefer
Denial	I can't believe. I can't understand.	It did happen. I can understand.
Overreacting	This is awful, horrible, unbearable.	This is unfortunate. How will it look in 5 years?
Always-Never Thinking	I will always feel sad, miserable, lonely. I will never succeed, achieve, be fulfilled.	These feelings will pass. Things can change. Many things are possible.
All or Nothing Thinking	I am, he is, you are totally incompetent, inconsiderate, rotten.	I can acknowledge a mistake and learn. I can find positive aspects of myself and others.
Mind Reading	He, she, they can perceive my inner tension, anxiety, nervousness.	Others rarely notice or concern themselves with with my inner state.

We have within our brains not only systems that perceive and react, but also systems that can observe and monitor the brain's activity.

all, why should we worry about other people's opinions when we consider how quickly these opinions can change?

We have examined six broad categories of self-talks that cause emotional tension. Anytime we are caught up in negative emotions, we can notice the self-talks that are causing and maintaining our distress and begin to change them.

This may seem difficult. Our old self-talks are familiar and hence credible. The revised and more reasonable self-talks may feel uncomfortable and falsely upbeat. But once we use them successfully, they will feel natural and will help us move through life with emotional balance.

AWARENESS AND MINDFULNESS

The process of awareness is based on the uniquely human capability of self-observation. We have within our brains not only systems that perceive and react, but also systems that can observe and monitor the brain's activity. This capacity is often very underdeveloped. But it is a capacity which can be strengthened.

The key element in awareness is noticing. We can pause in the flow of actions and reactions to observe our inner reality. But it is important not to judge what we notice. This tends to shut down the process of awareness. It is better to take several even, smooth diaphragmatic breaths, establish a moment of calmness, then notice our thoughts and feelings.

We can label our thoughts with simple descriptors such as "thoughts of the future" or "thoughts of the past." We can label the feelings as "anger," "sadness," "fear," or "disgust." We can notice how one thought is associated with another and how one feeling lies beneath another.

One good way to practice this technique is to take about five minutes each day, sit comfortably, breathe evenly, partially close the eyes, and then just observe the feelings that are present. You may notice layers of feelings, with some on top and readily apparent and others that emerge after a few minutes. Remember: Just notice the feelings. Don't react. Don't intervene. Notice the feelings, then let go of them.

With practice you will become skilled at mindfulness. You will feel more connected to your inner self. You will experience greater peace and calmness. With time and practice, you will be able to maintain self-awareness throughout the day.

DWELLING ON THE OPPOSITE

In the Yoga Sutras of Patanjali, an ancient text of yoga practices, a cognitive technique for reducing emotional tension known as *dwelling on the opposite* can be found. The idea is that when the mind is disturbed by feelings of anger, resentment, or anxiety, one encourages the opposite feelings.

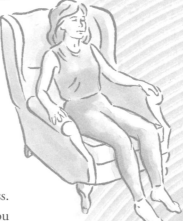

Take about five minutes each day, sit comfortably, breathe evenly, partially close the eyes, and then just observe the feelings that are present.

If you feel hatred toward someone, you could bring forth feelings of compassion and love for that person.

For example, if you feel anger toward someone, you might cultivate feelings of understanding toward that person. If you feel hatred toward someone, you could bring forth feelings of compassion and love for that person. If you feel disappointed in a family member, you can cultivate feelings of pride and appreciation.

The intent behind this technique is practical. The anger, hatred, and disappointment within only hurt you. Negative emotions spread like a cancer, stirring up more and more negative feelings. But when you create and dwell on the opposite feeling, you eliminate the negative emotions. You free yourself from emotional tension, calm your mind, and invite change.

To practice this technique, sit quietly and take a few even breaths. Close or partially close your eyes and become aware of the strong negative feelings you might have toward someone or some situation. Notice exactly what feelings you have and determine who or what they are directed against. Then simply begin to create the opposite feelings. Think positively of the person with whom you are upset. Think optimistically about the resolution of the conflict you face. For a few minutes, dwell on these new feelings.

At first this technique may seem simplistic. You may question the authenticity of your revised feelings and believe your anger feels more real. But this technique is about affecting your own freedom by letting go of judging others.

PHYSICAL APPROACHES TO EMOTIONAL RELAXATION

Breathing

The pattern of our breathing reflects our emotional state. When we are anxious, our inhalations are rapid and noisy. When we are afraid, we hold our breath. When we are depressed, we exhale with a long sigh. When we are startled, we gasp for breath and a shocking experience can literally knock the wind right out of us. And when we are tranquil, our breathing is smooth, even, and quiet.

The relationship between breathing and emotions is a two-way street. Our breathing pattern directly influences our emotional state. Establishing even, smooth diaphragmatic breathing creates a more balanced and peaceful emotional state.

Guidelines for the practice of even, smooth diaphragmatic breathing are provided in Chapter 5. This technique can be used at any time and in any place to quickly restore emotional balance. If you are arguing with another person and feel your temper flaring, you can start even, smooth diaphragmatic breathing and restore emotional balance. If you are feeling overwhelmed by a job, breathing diaphragmatically will help you regain energy and hope. If you are feeling anxious before a challenging

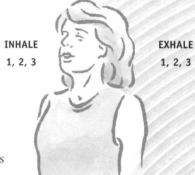

INHALE 1, 2, 3

EXHALE 1, 2, 3

The pattern of our breathing reflects our emotional state.

When you relax the facial muscles into a beginning smile and breathe evenly, you move toward a more relaxed state.

task, diaphragmatic breathing will calm you.

Diaphragmatic breathing can also prevent emotional tension. Practicing this technique for five or ten minutes at regular times during the day can help to maintain a balanced emotional state and prevent overreacting.

You can enhance the effects of diaphragmatic breathing by practicing "smile breathing." Once you establish smooth diaphragmatic breathing, let all of the tension out of your facial muscles and allow your face to settle into the beginning of a smile. Many negative emotions get patterned into facial tension. When you relax the facial muscles into a beginning smile and breathe evenly, you move toward a more relaxed state.

Working with your breathing will increase your awareness of your emotional nature. As you observe the relationship between breathing and feelings, you will experience emotional changes and reactions at more and more subtle levels.

EXERCISE AND MOVEMENT

Every emotional reaction organizes the body to move in a certain way. Conversely, different physical activities have direct and specific effects on our emotions.

We can use movement to release and express built-up emotions. Good examples of this are running, walking, rowing, aerobics, and biking, which help to express emotions such as fear and vigilance associated with the impulse for fleeing. Hard work and strenuous exercise often evaporate feelings of anger and aggression. Exercise gives us feelings of well-being and a sense of accomplishment.

MANAGING THE FOUR URGES

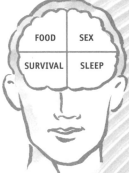

In the preceding chapter we learned that there were four basic urges or instinctual needs that profoundly influence our emotions: the urges for self-preservation, food, sleep, and sex. Much of our emotional life is based on our reactions to fulfilling or not fulfilling these four urges.

All too often the emotions generated by the four urges are negative. There may be brief interludes of happiness when we satisfy one or more of these urges. But typically we have emotional conflict about nourishment, safety and security, sleep and rest, and sexuality. A comprehensive approach to emotional relaxation requires that we learn to work with these four urges.

Managing the four urges involves four steps: knowledge, satisfaction, regulation, and mastery. The first, knowledge, has to do with studying and understanding the urge. The second step involves using this knowledge to satisfy the urge fully and remove conflict. Then we are in a

There may be brief interludes of happiness when we satisfy one or more of these urges.

When we are depressed, we sleep longer, have a hard time getting up, and are tired throughout the day.

position to regulate the urge with minimal risk of creating emotional conflict. Finally, with mastery we obtain freedom from the emotional pull of the urge.

In the case of the urge for food, we need to start with an understanding of the process of nourishment. Then we can choose a nourishing and satisfying diet. From this foundation we can regulate the urge for food without stirring up negative emotions. We can reduce what we eat or fast for a day without feeling anxious.

With mastery, we become free from emotional conflict based on the urge for food. We are happy when we have food, and happy when we don't.

In the case of the urge for sleep, most people, and particularly people with tension, rarely experience a good night's sleep. And without a good night's sleep, we are likely to feel irritable, anxious, deprived, and angry. Sleep and negative emotions are intertwined. When we are depressed, we sleep longer, have a hard time getting up, and are tired throughout the day. With anxiety, we have difficulty falling asleep, and we wake up throughout the night.

Sleep is the time when our body repairs and rebuilds from the demands of the day. Our mind rests, and emotional conflicts are resolved. Some cultures view sleep as a special time when our spiritual side reconnects with a spiritual source. Complete procedures for improving sleep are provided in Chapter 12, Relaxation in Daily Life.

The sexual urge is more complex because it involves a partner. Addressing the sexual urge demands that we understand not only the physiology of sex but also the nature of communication between partners. In order to obtain lasting and deepening sexual fulfillment with a partner, one must learn the art of communication and intimacy. Then it is possible to satisfy the sexual urge and enjoy such positive emotions as love, happiness, and joy while erasing worry, loneliness, and anxiety.

A couple can use communication to regulate their sexual life to avoid conflict and negative emotions. At the level of mastery, both preoccupation with sex and repression of sexual urges vanish.

The urge for self-preservation starts with protecting the physical self. The instinct for self-preservation is deeply ingrained, and when we feel threatened, fear arises. Once fear is locked into our emotional system, it becomes self-perpetuating. We see danger everywhere.

The same progression that we discussed with the other three urges applies to self-protection. The first step is knowledge of ourselves. We need to understand who we are. Then we can develop a belief in ourselves that makes us less vulnerable to fear.

We can overcome our fears by examining them to determine if they are realistic. We need to confront our fears

In order to obtain lasting and deepening sexual fulfillment with a partner, one must learn the act of communication and intimacy.

so they can fade away. We need to utilize self-talks as described earlier in the chapter to reduce our fears.

Sometimes the urge for self-preservation has more to do with protecting our ego. We worry about our status at work, our acceptance in the neighborhood, and respect from family members. Challenges to our ego lead to fear and anger.

Mastery of the urge for self-protection comes when our purpose is so clear, our knowledge of self so deep, and our wisdom so broad that we are fearless as we move forward in life.

TALKING AND LISTENING

Talk your feelings out in the presence of a good listener.

Emotional tension is most destructive when it is locked inside for months and years. Buried negative feelings have a corrosive effect on our emotional, physical, and mental life.

One of the simplest yet most effective ways to deal with these is to talk your feelings out in the presence of a good listener. If you are blessed with a friend or partner who can listen without reacting and judging, a friend in whose presence you feel secure and comfortable, then it will be quite helpful to air your worries, anxieties, and concerns.

Counseling can provide another opportunity to express feelings. An initial task of a therapist is to provide a space where you feel safe and comfortable expressing your feelings. A therapist can guide you to explore feelings and reactions that may have been beyond your conscious awareness. This releases deep emotional tension and enhances your self-awareness. A skilled therapist can help you to discover many ways to reduce emotional tension.

GUIDELINES FOR PRACTICE

The approaches to emotional relaxation described here can be applied both symptomatically and preventively. Some of the techniques, such as breathing and working with the self-talks, can help us manage an emotional crisis. Other techniques, such as awareness and exercise, can be used on a daily basis to change our patterns of emotional tension. Working with the four urges can be part of an overall lifestyle change to improve our emotional life.

If we feel angry or anxious, we can use the breathing techniques to stabilize our emotional state. Then we can examine our self-talks and change the thoughts that are upsetting us.

All the approaches to emotional relaxation are based on self-awareness. As we develop more awareness of our emotional responses and employ the methods of emotional relaxation, we will experience greater peace and tranquillity. We will be ready for the next step: relaxing the mind.

Working with the four urges can be part of an overall lifestyle change to improve our emotional life.

the mind
and mental
tension

O ur mind is housed in the brain where millions of neurons, myriad neurotransmitters, and a variety of brain systems and structures give us the capacity to think, perceive, will, feel, and remember. We even have the capability to be aware of these operations and to direct and manage them.

On an experiential level, our mind is our most constant and most personal companion. The instant we awaken, we begin thinking, perceiving, and remembering. Our thoughts can move from wishes for more sleep, to concerns about what we have to do during the day, to recollections of what happened yesterday. At the same time, our mind is rapidly perceiving, cataloging, and evaluating all kinds of sensory input. We might hear birds singing, smell the aroma of coffee, and see morning sunlight shining on the wall.

We can use our mind to accomplish incredible feats of learning, exploring, and creating. Our mind helps us solve the problems of everyday life and to fashion inventions and creations that can transform the future. With our mind, we can probe the secrets of nature, explore the mysteries of the past, and ponder the course of the future. Our mind enables us to communicate across distance and time through speech, print, music, and images.

But sometimes there seems to be no escape from the mind's activity. At the end of the day as we try to drift off to sleep, our mind is still running at breakneck speed, still

When we try to sleep, worries take over our mind and deny us the rest we crave.

processing thoughts, images, and memories, still noticing every sound. We worry about family and friends. We fret about past mistakes and feel guilt and remorse that can't be pushed away. We doubt our own worth and effectiveness. We worry about our physical health. We are anxious about the future.

No matter how often we distract ourselves with TV shows, movies, and games, our busy mind remains with us. No matter how much we intoxicate, stimulate, or stupefy the mind with drugs and alcohol, our worries remain with us. When we are alone, our concerns surface. When we try to sleep, worries take over our mind and deny us the rest we crave. At these times it seems our mind has become our enemy, an ever-present barrier to peace and tranquillity.

The mind is also the control room that creates tension on all the other levels of the body. Consider the all too common tension headache. It starts when our mind is filled with thoughts of too much work to do and not enough time to do it. As these thoughts reverberate through our mind, we feel more and more anxious, helpless, and even angry. These emotions create havoc in the autonomic nervous system. Blood pressure climbs, breathing becomes more rapid, and the blood vessels in the hands constrict, forcing more blood to the head. At the same time, the muscles of the shoulders, neck, and face tighten and brace as we automatically prepare for action. With all this commotion going on, it is just a matter of time until we have a pounding headache.

MENTAL TENSION

Mental tension creates two distinct conditions: the scattered, distracted, and unfocused mind; and the stuck and preoccupied mind.

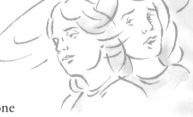

SCATTERED

The scattered mind's thoughts skip from one subject to the next. Externally, we are distracted by noises, sights, sensations, and even the smells around us. Internally, memories, ideas, plans, and fantasies jump into our mind. We can't stay focused.

The stuck mind replays the same thoughts over and over again. We keep seeing and hearing a rerun of an argument with a friend or family member. We might have some specific anxiety about the future that we can't get out of our head. We might have the same negative thoughts about our self echoing through our mind like a broken record.

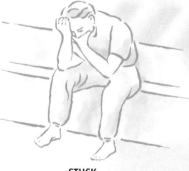

STUCK

When our mind is stuck, perception gets stuck. A certain irritating sound—a clock ticking, a dog barking, or a neighbor's stereo—might get stuck in our mind and grate on our nerves. We may feel the air is too warm or too cold,

When our mind is scattered and stuck, we fail to notice the world around us.

and keep thinking about it. There may be a smell in the environment that we can't ignore.

Most of the time, our thinking is both scattered and stuck. While we rehash an argument over and over in the foreground, in the background our thoughts skip through all the things we need to do. Or we can be consumed by worry, yet distracted by every sound and sight around us.

The tension created by the scattered and stuck mind leads to a number of problems. First of all, we lose awareness of the present. Our mind bounces back and forth between images and thoughts of the past and worries and concerns about the future. As mental tension increases, we often escape into fantasy, away from present reality.

Mental tension narrows our perception. When our mind is scattered and stuck, we fail to notice the world around us. We don't hear what people say.

Mental tension also acts to distort our perceptions. When we are upset, we may be blind to information that presents another view, deaf to words that tell another side of the story.

Mental tension also affects memory. We can't recall information we know is in our memory. We can't associate, organize, or categorize new information in a deep way. Ultimately, mental tension has a harmful effect on reasoning and problem solving. When our mind is anchored in the past or flying into the future, we don't have the data and resources we need for clear thinking. We are likely to make impulsive and unwise decisions.

THE RELAXED MIND

There are four essential qualities of the relaxed mind. First, a relaxed mind is centered. Instead of racing from thought to thought, the mind rests on one thought or one perception at a time. Then we can focus deeply on that thought or perception.

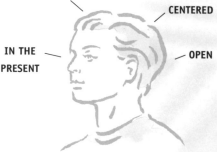

Second, the relaxed mind is open. When we are able to let go of worries and concerns, our thinking and perception become fresh and unbiased. We process the reactions and behavior of the people around us. We are fully aware of our own thoughts, feelings, and reactions and are open to our own true nature.

Third, the relaxed mind is nonjudgmental. We notice the thoughts and feelings that trace across our consciousness, but we don't get caught up in reacting to them. We don't judge one thought as good and another as bad. The relaxed mind can observe without reacting.

Finally, the relaxed mind is fully in the present. We notice the sensations and perceptions of the present moment. We are fully aware of our current feelings and thoughts.

There are four essential qualities of the relaxed mind.

A relaxed mind is
like a calm lake.
There are no
winds of worry to
stir the surface.

These four qualities may sound simple, but in fact are seldom experienced. Even a few minutes of mental relaxation can be completely transforming.

To better understand the nature of mental relaxation, we can compare the mind to a lake. Mental tension is like a turbulent lake. Worry about daily problems creates waves. Powerful currents of guilt and conflict further stir up the water. The twin tributaries of anxieties about the past and the future muddy the lake even more. If you drop a pebble into this turbulent lake, the impact will not be noticed. In a similar fashion, many events are not noticed by the tense mind.

A relaxed mind is like a calm lake. There are no winds of worry to stir the surface. The only currents are pure springs of inspiration which feed the lake from deep within. The tributaries of memory and expectation are absorbed without turbulence.

If you drop a pebble into a calm lake, you will notice the splash. You will see the rings spread concentrically from the point of impact. And then the lake will return to a calm state.

A calm mind experiences life in a similar fashion. We are fully aware of events in our environment. We watch events arise and fade away. And then our mind returns to a calm, balanced state.

When our mind is relaxed, reasoning and decision-making improve. We are better able to perceive the crucial data, to analyze a problem from all sides, and to problem solve effectively. When our mind is quiet, latent mental capacities emerge. We have more immediate and direct knowledge of things. We have access to our considerable intuitive powers. Creativity flows naturally. We get accurate hunches and strong feelings that elevate our problem-solving skills to new levels.

Mental relaxation also has a beneficial impact on all other levels of the body-mind. When our mind is quiet, we feel more peaceful and joyful. Our autonomic nervous system comes into balance. Our muscles relax.

Unfortunately, most of us have few experiences with a relaxed mind. At best we can recall a few instances when our mind was truly calm. It might have been a moment sitting on a deserted beach, absorbed in the sound of the wind and waves and watching the flow of the surf. Or it may have been a moment when we were absorbed in some creative art or craft project. Briefly our mind was calm and free of worries.

We can learn to create a relaxed mind. When we consider that the mind determines how we experience life, we realize that achieving mental relaxation should be a priority in our lives.

When our mind is quiet, latent mental capacities emerge.

chapter nine

Level IV:
mental relaxation

techniques

T here are three major approaches to mental relaxation: sensory focusing, concentration, and meditation.

SENSORY FOCUSING

As outlined in the previous chapter, when our mind is relaxed, we are aware of the sights, sounds, and sensations around us. Consequently, we can achieve mental relaxation by focusing on specific sensory input. We can use perception as a tool to bring our mind into the present.

Consider what happens when you are driving in the country and see a spectacular sunset. You immediately forget your cares. Your mind is cleared of worries, and feelings of joy overcome you. A beautiful piece of music on the car radio could have the same impact.

Unfortunately, such experiences are infrequent. Usually we glance at a sunset, but don't really see it. And the music is drowned out by mental tension's inner chatter.

In each instance, perception offered the opportunity to bring our awareness into the present, but the pull of mental tension was too strong. However, we can learn to use perception to bring our awareness into the present. We can select some sight, sound, or simple daily activity, focus on it, and bring our awareness into the present.

The key is to notice without judging or reacting. As we open to sensory input, our mind comes into the present, our breathing slows, and the muscles in our face, neck, and shoulders relax. Our emotions calm.

A good beginning sensory focusing technique is called the *Circle of Sound*.

the practice

Imagine you are at the center of a clock and the numbers on the clock face represent all the directions around you.

- This technique can be practiced either inside a room or outside in a natural setting. It can be practiced in a quiet space or a noisy environment.
- Begin by sitting in a comfortable chair or stretching out on the floor or the ground. Take a few minutes to let go of any tension in your face and throughout your body. Make your breathing even, smooth, and diaphragmatic.
- Picture yourself at the center of a circle of sound. If it helps, you can imagine you are at the center of a clock and the numbers on the clock face represent all the directions around you.
- Notice the sounds in your environment. Notice the location of any sound. Locate it on your clock. A sound might move across from one point to another.
- Describe the quality of the sound to yourself. Does it have a high pitch or a low pitch? Is it constant or changing?

Is there one sound or more? Is it rhythmic or irregular? Is it mechanical or natural?

- Describe the sound. Try to avoid judging, analyzing, or reacting to it. If your mind drifts away to some associations or memories, just bring your awareness back to the Circle of Sound. Keep scanning it to discover any new sounds that emerge or subtle sounds you didn't hear at first.

- Practice this technique for five to ten minutes. When the time is up, take a few deep breaths, open your eyes, and notice how clear and refreshed your mind is.

CONCENTRATION

Concentration is the process of directing attention toward a single object. During the practice of concentration, the mind is focused on one thing rather than jumping from object to object. Just as a scattered and distracted mind indicates tension, a centered and focused mind is a sign of relaxation.

The idea that concentration leads to relaxation may seem surprising. Usually when we think of concentration, we think of effort and work. When we hear the word "concentrate," we might hear the echo of a parent's or a teacher's voice urging us to "concentrate" on our homework. Concentration felt like hard work for our young

A centered and focused mind is a sign of relaxation.

mind. In reality, it takes more mental energy to jump from thought to thought.

If our mind is in the habit of jumping from subject to subject, it will take some training and effort for us to sustain concentration. We need to go easy at first. We don't want to force ourselves and create more mental stress.

The following concentration exercise starts with the breath as a point of focus. Even, smooth diaphragmatic breathing provides a rhythmic and soothing object of concentration. You can either read through and memorize these instructions or record them.

Bend your knees so that your feet rest flat on the floor directly beneath them.

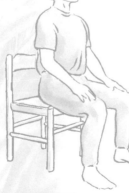

CONCENTRATION ON THE BREATH

the practice

- In a quiet and comfortable room, sit on the front edge of a firm chair. Bend your knees so that your feet rest flat on the floor directly beneath them. Adjust your posture. Bring your shoulders back. Allow a natural curve in your lower back. Align your head so that your ears are above your shoulders and your lower back. Your gaze should be straight ahead.

- Close your eyes. Exhale completely and allow a deep inhalation to follow. Repeat this two times. Let your breath settle into a smooth, even diaphragmatic pattern.

- Now begin a brief muscular relaxation. Bring your awareness to both hands and let go of any extra tension. Soften and relax the muscles in the hands. Move your awareness to your wrists and lower arms, and let go and lengthen the muscles in your lower arms.
- Let go in your upper arms and shoulders. Let go across your chest, down the sides of your torso, and across your abdomen. Guide your awareness to the pelvis and let go of unneeded tension. Release through the hips and upper legs. Let go around your knees, calves, shins, and ankles. Guide your attention to your feet, and soften and lengthen the muscles on the top and bottom of each foot. Relax all ten toes.
- Bring your awareness to your lower back and release any tension there. Let go up and down the back on both sides of the spine. Let go around your shoulder blades and up into the back of your neck. Soften and lengthen the muscles all around your neck. Let go across the back of your head, top of your head, and your forehead. Release around the eyes, across the jaw muscles, around the lips and chin.
- Now bring your attention back to your breathing. Establish even, smooth diaphragmatic breath. As you exhale, your abdomen is smoothly contracted. As you inhale, relax your abdomen and feel the breath flow deeply into your lungs. Make the inhalation and exhalation the same length. Keep the flow of your breath

smooth. Eliminate any jerks and halts.

- Now begin to focus your mind on the inhalation and exhalation. As the breath flows in, notice the sensation of the air through your nostrils. That air flow may feel cool and dry. Then notice the sensation of the air as it flows out with your exhalation. That air may feel warm and moist.

- Direct your attention entirely to your breathing, to the inhalations and the exhalations. Feel the cooler, dryer air flowing in and the warmer, moister air flowing out. You can think to yourself, "Cool, dry air in; warm, moist air out." Keep your attention on the pattern and sensation of your breathing.

- If some distraction disrupts your concentration, just let go of the distraction and bring your attention back to the inhalations and exhalations, to the sensation of the cool, dry air in and the warm, moist air out. Reestablish your concentration, redirect your attention to the flow of the breath.

- Keep the experience easy and comfortable. Check the muscles in your face to make sure there is no sense of struggle or striving creeping in. Loosen the muscles in your forehead, around your eyes, across the jaw, and through the lower face. Keep your breathing even, smooth, diaphragmatic, and slow.

- Focus on your breathing for a comfortable interval of time. At the beginning, this may be five to ten minutes. Later, as you increase your capacity, you will be able to

Check the muscles in your face to make sure there is no sense of struggle or striving creeping in.

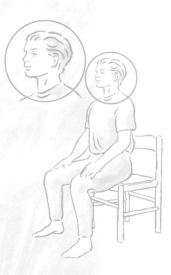

sustain concentration for twenty minutes or more.

- When you have finished your session of concentration, take a few deeper breaths. Direct your awareness to your arms and legs. Gently move your hands and feet. Bring your hands up to cover your eyes. Open your eyes behind your hands, and bring your hands away, returning your awareness to the world around you.

- Take a moment to reflect on your inner state. Keep awareness of the relaxed mind with you as you resume your day's activities.

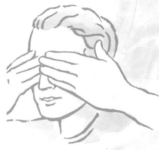

MEDITATION

"Meditation" is an English approximation for the Sanskrit word *dhyana*, which means an unbroken flow of thought toward an object of concentration. The object of meditation might be a word, a picture, an image, a concept, or the breath. If the object of meditation is a word, you start by concentrating on that word. As your concentration deepens, your mind flows continually toward this word. As you move deeper into meditation, your mind becomes totally absorbed in that word.

During meditation, the thinking process is stilled. The mind becomes quiet, providing profound rest for the mind, with the result that it returns to thought refreshed and

Open your eyes behind your hands, and bring your hands away, returning your awareness to the world around you.

**Meditation is the
finest method for
creating mental
relaxation.**

revitalized. Meditation is the finest method for creating mental relaxation.

There are misunderstandings about meditation. Often when we hear the word, we think of the dictionary definition "to think deeply or ponder some subject." But here we are referring to a distinct process for working with the mind, not a type of thinking. Meditation is conscious effort to focus the mind in a nonanalytic manner and to move away from thinking about things.

Another misunderstanding arises from the association between meditation and mystical practices or an ascetic lifestyle. But meditation can be effectively practiced by people richly involved with life who want to experience optimal health and well-being.

Research studies have consistently shown that when people practice meditation, their psychological well-being improves. Meditators experience improved self-esteem, decreased anxiety and depression, higher levels of self-actualization, and better overall health.

the
practice

- The practice of meditation involves a number of systematic steps. We will explore each of these steps in order.

- First, choose a regular time for meditation. That way you don't have to make a decision each day, but will form a positive habit. Then your mind and body will spontaneously prepare for the practice of meditation.

- Generally, early in the morning, late in the afternoon, or in the evening before going to bed are suitable times for meditation. Many people prefer to get up a few minutes early to practice meditation, because the mind has not yet been flooded with impressions and the environment is quiet. It can also be quite helpful to clear the mind at the end of the workday or at night before bed.

- A specific place in your home or apartment should be set aside for meditation. Select a spot that is pleasant and quiet, has adequate fresh air, and isn't used for other purposes. A quiet corner of a room is fine. As time goes by, you will develop an association with this spot and it will feel quite natural to sit there and meditate.

- Second, preparation for meditation is important. The following guidelines should be seen not as fixed rules, but as steps that can improve the quality of meditation.

- Taking a shower or washing your face and hands beforehand will help you feel refreshed and purified. It is hard to meditate while your body is preoccupied with digesting food, so it is best to meditate before eating or after a light meal. You should wait several hours after a heavy meal.

Select a spot that is pleasant and quiet, has adequate fresh air, and isn't used for other purposes.

- Loose, comfortable clothing is most suitable for meditation. Remove glasses, watchband, hard contact lenses, or anything that puts pressure on your body. Take off your shoes. During meditation, respiration and metabolism slow and you will tend to cool off. It is a good idea to wear a warm shirt or sweatshirt, or to drape a shawl or light blanket over your shoulders.

- A few stretches or light exercises can help to loosen up your body and make it easier to sit for meditation. Some people find a brief walk before meditation is another helpful way to loosen up the muscles and smooth out the breathing. A short session of muscular relaxation can release tension and help prepare you for meditation.

- Third, the position or posture for meditation is important and should allow you to sit comfortably and steadily, with your head, neck, and trunk aligned. The posture should encourage alert attention and inner balance.

- One suitable position is to sit in a firm chair as described in the section on concentration. This posture, called *the friendship pose,* can be comfortably performed by a person of any age or level of fitness.

- Another good posture for meditation is called *the easy pose.* This posture involves sitting on the floor and crossing your legs in front of you so that the left knee rests on the right foot and the right knee rests on the left foot. A firm cushion under your buttocks will make it easier to assume the natural S curve in your back and you will sit more comfortably. Once you have aligned your head, neck, and trunk, you can place your palms on your knees.

- *The auspicious pose* is more challenging and requires greater flexibility. In this pose, the legs are brought in closer to the body and the knees extended out farther, creating a firm and steady base. Sit on the floor, bend your right leg at the knee and place the sole of your right foot against your right thigh. Then bring your left ankle under your right ankle and position the sole of your left foot against your right thigh. Both feet should be positioned so only the big toe is seen. Place a firm cushion or a folded blanket under your buttocks to increase the comfort of the position and to create a natural curve in your lower back. Then align your head, neck, and trunk.

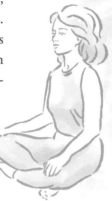

EASY POSE

- The last step is to choose an object of meditation. Within the various traditions of meditation are many choices. *Mantras* are words or sounds that can be repeated over and over. *Yantras* are geometric forms designed to represent positive states of consciousness. There are prayers that can be used for meditation. Meditating on the breath is a good technique for beginners. This is a method emphasized in the Zen Buddhist tradition.

AUSPICIOUS POSE

OVERCOMING OBSTACLES

The practice of meditation sounds simple and seems straightforward. Yet as we meditate, we may encounter obstacles and distractions. One obstacle may be our own tendency to strive and push for results. If we force ourselves to focus, we may increase tension.

In meditation, less effort brings more results. All we need to do in meditation is to quiet the mind. When this stillness is achieved, many things are accomplished. The nervous system moves to a state of balance, and the body rests. In stillness, we access deeper levels of self, which nourishes our spirit.

Obstacles can come from the thoughts that enter our mind during meditation. We might notice sounds and smells in our environment. We might notice discomfort in our body. These distractions are very common. They often generate a string of thoughts and feelings that pull us away from the object of meditation.

Sometimes physical discomforts are manifestations of mental restlessness. The mind resists our efforts to focus it by seizing on some minor itch or ache and magnifying it until we are overwhelmed by discomfort. If you find this happening, label the precise discomfort dispassionately and return your awareness to the object of meditation. Usually the discomfort will disappear.

In meditation, less effort brings more results.

The best way to deal with mental distractions is to gently bring your attention back to the object of meditation. Avoid becoming impatient. Simply notice the distraction, let go, and return your awareness to the object of meditation. If the distracting thoughts persist, you can label them in a nonjudgmental way. Classify each distraction as a thought about the past or the future.

Categorizing distracting thoughts allows us to witness them in an objective manner. We don't have to suppress them; we can simply notice them, and let go. Gradually our mind will calm, distractions will come less frequently, and our meditation will deepen.

As we quiet the mind, innovative ideas and creative solutions may emerge. We should let go of these ideas. If we thought of them once, they will come back when we need them. Learn to regard "great ideas" with the same equanimity with which you view negative reactions. Let go and return your awareness to the breath.

Occasionally as we meditate, a vivid memory of a traumatic event may come into our consciousness. We may respond with strong emotions to this memory. We may react, judge, or try to analyze it. The emergence of suppressed material may be a sign that meditation is helping to cleanse and purify the mind. As with all other distractions, we can just witness the event, notice our response, and then return our awareness to the breath.

Learn to regard "great ideas" with the same equanimity with which you view negative reactions.

Any time you let go of a distraction and return your attention to your breathing or another object of meditation, check your meditation posture. Make sure that your head, neck, and trunk are aligned, that the facial muscles are relaxed and smooth, and that your breathing is smooth. Allow a trace of a beginning smile to come into your face. Let go of any holding in the shoulders and neck.

Sometimes meditation is surprising. When we feel clear and focused, we may anticipate a serene session of meditation only to discover chaos within. On other days when we are so stressed out that we have to push ourselves to meditate, we may quickly find great calmness and silence within. It is best to be free of expectations.

The effects of meditation are cumulative. Each time we meditate, we establish a pathway in the mind. With each session, this pathway becomes deeper and smoother, allowing us greater access to the meditative state.

ENCOURAGING MEDITATION

There are a number of things you can do to help encourage daily meditative practice. First of all, if you make meditation pleasant and enjoyable, you will want to do it more.

Secondly, you need to have a degree of commitment and self-discipline. Make a personal commitment to meditate on a daily basis. Start with a commitment to meditate for thirty days. Set aside twenty minutes of your day for meditation. You may notice that you actually gain time by requiring less sleep and by being more alert and productive during the day.

Inspiration can help you to maintain this commitment. There are many books from the various meditative traditions that describe the compelling personal experiences of dedicated individuals who have followed the path of meditation. Reading these books can energize and strengthen your resolve to meditate. Learning more about additional breathing, concentration, and meditative approaches can deepen your practice.

You can also strengthen your meditation by practicing "meditation in action." As you drive your car, wash the dishes, mow the lawn, talk to a business partner, or do paperwork, keep part of your attention centered on the object of meditation. This acts as a calming anchor for the mind. This helps you to maintain continuity and connection with the meditative state. It brings a sense of balance and peacefulness into everyday life.

A guided meditation practice is on the CD accompanying this book.

You can also strengthen your meditation by practicing "meditation in action."

chapter ten

the

spiritual

level

S pirituality is at once the most compelling level of human experience and yet the most challenging to describe and define. Spiritual concerns are a central part of life, yet there is no readily identifiable physiological location where our spiritual sensibilities reside. But in our hearts and minds we know that the spiritual dimension of life is important and real.

WHAT IS SPIRITUALITY?

What persistent themes run through the spiritual life of humankind? First, there is belief in an aspect of life that lies beyond the ordinary, beyond daily events, beyond that which can be measured and weighed—a sacred dimension.

This sacred dimension is seen to be imbued with qualities that influence and direct the course of daily events. Some cultures believe that spiritual forces bring the rain, the wind, the sun, and the seasons. In Hindu cultures it is felt that various gods and goddesses influence specific aspects of life such as agriculture, war, business, love, or politics. In monotheistic religions, spiritual power resides in an ultimate being known as God. God is viewed as transcendent yet intimately involved in human affairs.

Some religious practices include rituals to curry favor with and appease spiritual forces in the environment. Shamans enter trance states to receive direct spiritual

A code of moral
behavior is part of
most spiritual
traditions.

guidance. Many religions offer sacrifices to invite the favorable intervention of a specific god. More familiar to western society is development of a relationship with god.

A code of moral behavior is part of most spiritual traditions. In the Old Testament, Moses gave his people the Ten Commandments to help them distinguish right from wrong.

Spiritual traditions also are concerned with the development of human potential. Scriptures often present an image and an ideal on how to become a complete person and fulfill one's purpose in life. Most spiritual traditions also present a story of creation, of how the world began. And spiritual traditions help people to understand and cope with death.

SPIRITUAL TENSION

Spiritual tension is the most subtle, yet ultimately the most damaging, kind of tension. It creates deep conflict in the mind, persistent negative emotions, and tension in the nervous system. Spiritual tension dwells at the core of our being, weakens our ability to cope, and diminishes our vitality and creativity.

The primary symptoms of tension on the spiritual level are feelings of disconnection, alienation, emptiness, and isolation. Life has little meaning, pleasures are fleeting, and there is nothing to look forward to with expectation. Life becomes a matter of putting in time.

Spiritual tension leads to cynicism. We begin to believe immediate self-interest is the only motivating force in people. We may seize on this same principle of self-interest as our own primary motivation. We become disillusioned with civic and social institutions. We find it difficult to believe in anything.

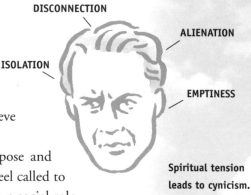

Spiritual tension leads to cynicism.

Disillusionment leads to a lack of purpose and direction in life. Consequently, we will not feel called to any role in life, whether that is a family role, a social role, a religious role, or a vocational role.

Without a spiritual perspective, we may lack a set of ethical and behavioral guidelines to support our personal conscience. We may ascribe to the belief that there is no real right or wrong, and behave with only self-interest as our guide.

Without the reinforcement and encouragement of a spiritual path, we may end up behaving in ways that conflict with our core values. Over time, feelings of guilt can accumulate deep in our psyche.

When there is tension on the spiritual level, we are cut off from guidance from a higher level. We will not have spiritual input to help us make difficult decisions, to support us through rough times, or to guide us in choosing the best path of personal development.

SPIRITUAL RELAXATION

Spiritual relaxation involves more than reducing tension. It is integrative and positive. It comes only through direct spiritual experience. Spiritual experiences are based on and encourage faith and belief. As faith and belief grow, we are able to participate in spiritual practices such as prayer and worship. We can organize our lives around ethical guidelines and embrace a system that encourages development to our highest potential. We will have a belief system to help us understand and cope with our death and the deaths of those we love.

There are many types of spiritual experiences, ranging from a moment of peace during worship to a transcendent instant while viewing the beauty of nature. Spiritual experiences can come in dreams, in prayer, through fellowship, through song, through the reading and study of sacred scriptures, or through contemplation and meditation. These experiences give us communication and interaction with a power or spirit that is both beyond and within ourselves.

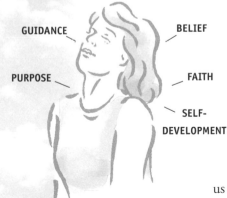

Spiritual relaxation involves more than reducing tension.

GUIDANCE

PURPOSE

BELIEF

FAITH

SELF-
DEVELOPMENT

In some traditional cultures, periods of solitary fasting, meditation, and intense prayer would open one to a vision during which spiritual guidance would be received. Such experiences deepen our awareness of a greater pattern and deeper dimension of life. Our lives take on a larger meaning. We feel a connection to the spiritual core of life, a sense of connection which overcomes feelings of isolation and helplessness. We have a feeling of being supported and helped on the journey of life.

Another dimension of spiritual relaxation is the emergence of a sense of purpose and direction in our life. We sense we have a role to play, a job to complete, and duties to perform. As we progress in our spiritual growth, we may feel inspired to achieve goals, to take on specific challenges, to address problems or injustices that exist in the world. With spiritual integration, we understand that we are fulfilling a destiny greater than ourselves.

Internalizing practical, ethical guidelines strengthens our conscience, giving us a clear sense of right and wrong. As we live in accordance with these guidelines, our will becomes strong. Our mind and emotions are not weakened by conflict.

THE EFFECTS OF SPIRITUAL RELAXATION

People with strong spiritual beliefs have been found to cope

Individuals with strong spiritual beliefs suffer less from depression and anxiety.

better with both major and minor stressful events. They are more resilient. They seem to feel supported as they cope with life's difficulties. They are better able to view difficult situations as a call for spiritual growth.

Spiritual relaxation has a beneficial effect on emotional well being. Individuals with strong spiritual beliefs suffer less from depression and anxiety. A spiritually oriented lifestyle has a positive impact on physical health, decreasing blood pressure, cardiovascular disease, and cancer. These benefits are most apparent when people perceive the spiritual realm as a source of love and compassion.

Spiritual relaxation energizes the process of self-actualization. People with a spiritual outlook are less likely to be preoccupied with physiological and safety needs, as they have faith that their needs will be met. This frees them to dedicate themselves to ideals and purposes outside themselves.

Spiritual relaxation increases the likelihood of having what the noted psychologist Abraham Maslow called *peak experiences.* These are moments of spiritual integration, clarity, and awareness. During a peak experience the transcendent and sacred nature of life is revealed, and the unity behind the complexity and contradictions of life is perceived. Peak experiences energize the self-development process.

Peak experiences dramatically verify the reality of the

spiritual level. They strengthen belief and faith. They change one's perspective of one's self and of the nature of the world. These experiences open one to deeper spiritual perspective.

The effects of spiritual relaxation and integration are profound. Spiritual relaxation operates at the most subtle level, yet directly influences all the other levels. Let us now explore the various approaches to spiritual relaxation.

During a peak experience the transcendent and sacred nature of life is revealed.

chapter eleven

Level V:
spiritual relaxation
techniques

S piritual relaxation comes through direct and meaningful experience of the sacred. The methods described below are common to many religions and spiritual traditions. The format and content of each method may differ, but the intent of interacting with the spiritual level remains the same.

WORSHIP

Worship is the highest expression of faith and devotion. Worship is at the core of every religion. It can mean attending a service at a church, temple, or mosque. Or it can mean daily practice before a shrine in your home

In organized religion, worship takes place within the context of a developed theology and creed. Worship can include the study of sacred scripture, the giving of offerings, and participation in sacraments. Worship involves honoring the Divine. This may occur in the form of words or songs, or it may be carried out through actions performed in a spirit of devotion. Prayer is often a major component.

Worship typically occurs at a specific time. This could be on a weekly basis as in a Protestant Sunday service or a Jewish Sabbath. Or worship can occur at regular times during the day, as it does for Muslims. It can be formal and structured, as in a Catholic Mass, or informal and free-flowing, as in a prayer meeting. Worship can be in public or in private.

Our prayers should be offered with single-minded attention, in a spirit not of expectation, but of trust, belief, and devotion.

Worship is the broadest category of spiritual experience. It contains all the methods discussed below. Everyone has the opportunity to make worship a priority in his or her life, to devote time each day or week to the spiritual path, and to enhance the process of spiritual relaxation.

PRAYER

Prayer is a fundamental part of every religion and spiritual tradition. The word "pray" comes from the Latin word meaning "to ask." To pray is to ask. It is also a way for us to open ourselves to humility and compassion.

There are many forms of prayer. There are prayers of thanksgiving and adoration. There are prayers of confession. And there are prayers of petition where we ask for help with our own needs. This may include prayers asking for health, material benefits, or such personal qualities as courage, compassion, or grace. We may petition for divine guidance to help us make important life decisions. We may also ask for intercession on behalf of others.

Of particular importance is the manner in which we pray. Our prayers should be offered with single-minded attention, in a spirit not of expectation, but of trust, belief, and devotion. It is not enough to just repeat the words of a prayer. St. Augustine, an early father of the Christian church, wrote, "True prayer is nothing but love."

Belief is also important. In the New Testament, Jesus spoke on this: "I tell you whatever you ask for in prayer, believe that you have received it, and it will be yours." In other words, the stronger the belief, the more powerful the prayer.

The effects of prayer have been receiving increased attention from scientists and health care practitioners. Dr. Larry Dossey, the author of two books on the role of prayer in healing and medicine, notes that there are over 130 scientific studies that show the beneficial effects of prayer. In one of these studies a group of prayed-for coronary patients showed greater improvement than those who weren't prayed for. In controlled laboratory experiments, prayer had beneficial effects on baby gerbils, germinating seeds, rats, mice, bacteria, and fungi.

These studies suggest that prayer operates across distance and through space and that the spiritual domain is entirely unique. Unlike the material world where the principle of cause-and-effect operates, something far more subtle seems to be at work in the spiritual dimension. Clearly, the spirit in which a prayer is made influences the effect it has. Prayers offered with compassion, empathy, and love are the most powerful.

Studies suggest that prayer operates across distance and through space and that the spiritual domain is entirely unique.

the
practice

Prayer can be practiced standing, sitting, walking, or kneeling. A sitting or kneeling position facilitates stillness and focusing. A standing position implies an attitude of honor and respect. Bending the head forward expresses humility. Prayers can be spoken aloud, subvocalized, or offered in silence.

Below are prayers from different spiritual traditions of the world. These prayers can be repeated daily or included in regular worship. Some of them fill us with feelings of peace and serenity. Others offer protection and guidance. Some inspire compassion and hope; some strengthen our sense of purpose.

Peace and Serenity

May the peace of God, which passes all understanding, keep your hearts and minds in the knowledge and love of God, and of his son Jesus Christ our Lord. And the blessing of God almighty, the Father, Son, and Holy Ghost, be among you and with you always.

—Book of Common Prayer[7]

7. Patrick Cotter, *How to Pray* (Boca Raton: Globe Communications Corp., 1996), 63.

God, grant me the serenity to accept the things
    I cannot change;
courage to change the things I can; and wisdom to
    know the difference.
Living one day at a time;
Enjoying one moment at a time;
Accepting hardships as the pathway to peace;
Taking this sinful world as it is, not as I would have it;
Trusting that you will make all things right if I
    surrender to your will;
That I may be reasonably happy in this life
And supremely happy with you forever in the next.
              —Attributed to Reinhold Niebuhr[8]

May there be peace in the higher regions; may there
be peace in the firmament; may there be peace on
earth. May the waters flow peacefully; may the herbs
and plants grow peacefully; may all the divine powers
bring unto us peace. The supreme Lord is peace. May
we all be in peace, peace, and only peace; and may
that peace come unto each of us.

                    —The Vedas[9]

8. David Schiller, ed., *The Little Book of Prayers* (New York: Workman Publishing, 1996), 316.

9. George Appleton, ed., *The Oxford Book of Prayer* (New York: Oxford University Press, 1985), 285.

Guidance

Lord, make me an instrument of your peace.
Where there is hatred, let me sow love,
Where there is injury, pardon;
Where there is doubt, faith;
Where there is despair, hope;
Where there is darkness, light;
Where there is sadness, joy.

O Divine Master, grant that I may not so much
    seek to be consoled as to console,
    to be understood as to understand,
    to be loved, as to love.

For it is in giving that we receive,
    it is in pardoning that we are pardoned,
    and it is in dying that we are born to eternal life.

—St. Francis of Assisi[10]

Lead me from the unreal to the Real.
Lead me from darkness to Light.
Lead me from death to Immortality.
Om, Peace, Peace, Peace

—Upanishads[11]

10. Schiller, ed., *The Little Book of Prayers*, 192.

11. Yogiraj Sri Swami Satchidananda, *Integral Yoga Hatha* (New York: Holt, Rinehart and Winston, 1970), xxix.

O our Father the Sky, hear us and make us bold.

O our Mother the Earth, hear us and give us support.

O Spirit of the East, send us your wisdom.

O Spirit of the South, may we walk your path of life.

O Spirit of the West, may we always be ready for the
long journey.

O Spirit of the North, purify us with your cleansing
winds.

—Sioux Prayer[12]

Protection and Support

The Lord is my shepherd; I shall not want.

He makes me to lie down in green pastures;

He leads me beside the still waters.

He restores my soul; He leads me in the paths of
righteousness for His name's sake.

Yea, though I walk through the valley of the
shadow of death, I will fear no evil;
for You are with me;

Your rod and Your staff, they comfort me.

You prepare a table before me in the presence
of my enemies;

You anoint my head with oil;

My cup runs over.

12. Schiller, ed., *The Little Book of Prayers*, 204.

Surely goodness and mercy shall follow me
 All the days of my life;
And I will dwell in the house of the Lord
Forever.

        —Twenty-third Psalm[13]

Protect me, O Lord;
My boat is so small, And your sea is so big.

        —The Fishermen's Prayer[14]

Now that evening has fallen,
To God, the Creator, I will turn in prayer,
Knowing that he will help me.
I know the Father will help me.

        —Dinka, Sudan[15]

Belief and Faith

I believe in the sun even when it is not shining.
I believe in love even when feeling it not.
I believe in God even when he is silent.

        —Jewish Prayer[16]

13. *The New King James Bible, New Testament* (Nashville: Thomas Nelson Publishers, 1980), 510.

14. Barbara Greene and Victor Gollancz, *God of a Hundred Names* (New York: Doubleday & Company, 1962), 69.

15. Appleton, ed., *The Oxford Book of Prayer,* 351.

16. Schiller, ed., *The Little Book of Prayers,* 308.

God is the Eternal One, he is everlasting and is without end. He is everlasting and eternal. He endureth for time without end, and he will exist to all eternity.

—Old Egyptian[17]

O Thou who art at home
Deep in my heart
Enable me to join you
Deep in my heart.

—The Talmud[18]

Praise and Thanksgiving

Blessed art thou, O Lord our God, King of the Universe, who createst thy world every morning afresh.

—Contemporary Hebrew Prayer[19]

God is the light of the heavens and the earth. His light may be compared to a niche that enshrines a lamp, the lamp within a crystal of star-like brilliance. It is lit from a blessed olive tree neither eastern nor western. Its very oil would almost shine forth, though no fire touched it. Light upon light; God guides to His light whom He will.

17. Greene and Gollancz, *God of a Hundred Names*, 271.
18. Schiller, ed., *The Little Book of Prayers*, 195.
19. Greene and Gollancz, *God of a Hundred Names*, 19.

God speaks in parables to mankind. God has knowledge of all things.

—Koran from Sura XXIV[20]

With your feet I walk
I walk with your limbs
I carry forth your body
For me your mind thinks
Your voice speaks for me
Beauty is before me
And beauty is behind me
Above and below me hovers the beautiful
I am surrounded by it
I am immersed in it
In my youth I am aware of it
And in my old age I shall walk quietly
The beautiful trail.

—Navajo Prayer[21]

Earth our mother, breathe forth life
    all night sleeping
    now awaking
    in the east
    now see the dawn
Earth our mother, breathe and waken

20. N. J. Dawood, trans., *The Koran* (New York: Penguin Books, 1997), 249.
21. Schiller, ed., *The Little Book of Prayers,* 21.

leaves are stirring
all things moving
new day coming
life renewing   —Pawnee Prayer[22]

Compassion

May all beings have happiness, and the causes
    of happiness;
May all be free from sorrow, and the causes of sorrow;
May all never be separated from the sacred happiness
    which is sorrowless;
And may all live in equanimity, without too much
    attachment and too much aversion,
And live believing in the equality of all that lives.
                      —Buddhist Prayer[23]

However innumerable beings are, I vow to save them;
However inexhaustible the passions are, I vow to
    extinguish them;
However immeasurable the Dharmas are, I vow to
    master them;
However incomparable the Buddha-truth is, I vow to
    attain it.
             —Zen Prayer After Meditation[24]

22. Schiller, ed., *The Little Book of Prayers,* 152.

23. Schiller, ed., *The Little Book of Prayers,* 121.

24. Appleton, ed., *The Oxford Book of Prayer,* 357.

Let the prayer flow
from your heart
in a spontaneous
fashion. Don't
worry about
getting the
wording right.

In addition to these structured prayers, you can make up your own prayer to offer thanksgiving, to ask for forgiveness, or to petition for help or guidance for yourself or for others. Let the prayer flow from your heart in a spontaneous fashion. Don't worry about getting the wording right. Just say the prayer in the present tense, concentrate on the meaning, and pray with full belief.

CONTEMPLATION

To "contemplate" means to look at attentively and thoughtfully, to consider carefully and at length. As a spiritual practice, contemplation is a method for reflecting on a religious truth in order to arrive at a personal understanding and love it for what it signifies.

A person might contemplate a line or passage of scripture. As one memorizes and repeats the phrase, one first attempts to grasp the meaning of the phrase, to understand it intellectually. As contemplation deepens, one's inner being, one's heart, and one's feelings are grasped by the deepest meaning of the phrase.

The word "contemplation" comes from the Latin root *con,* meaning "with" and *templum,* meaning "a space for observing auguries." In contemplation, we become a place where the spiritual level can be observed. We align our life with the sacred.

Different spiritual traditions have developed various types of contemplation. Within the Christian tradition, passages from the Bible, or icons of Christ or various saints are used as objects of contemplation.

In the spiritual exercises developed by St. Ignatius Loyola, a sixteenth-century mystic and missionary, the mind visualized an episode in the life of Christ. Employing all of the senses, one sees, hears, and feels the episode, entering the scene as a witness, then as a participant, filling one's mind and heart with it.

In the Tantric branch of Buddhism, aspirants contemplate complex geometric figures known as *mandalas.* These carefully constructed patterns of triangles, circles, and rectangles are designed to represent the sacred order of the cosmos. They are blueprints or diagrams for the spiritual dimension, a method of spiritual transformation. As one contemplates a mandala and becomes totally absorbed in it, one moves beyond a scientific, materialistic view of the world, beyond an intellectual understanding of the sacred, to a direct experience of it.

There is considerable latitude in choosing an object of contemplation. As mentioned above, a line of scripture, a philosophical thesis, an image of Christ, the words of a teacher are all suitable objects of contemplation. You simply need to take some quiet time, free from interruptions, and consider the object of contemplation.

A line of scripture, a philosophical thesis, an image of Christ, the words of a teacher are all suitable objects of contemplation.

MEDITATION

In Chapter 9 we discussed meditation as a method for easing mental tension. But meditation can also be a profoundly spiritual practice. While contemplation approaches the sacred by filling the mind and heart with an image of the ideal, meditation quiets and empties the mind and thereby opens the self to the imprint of the sacred. In meditation, when we quiet the thinking process and calm the emotions, the mind and heart become a spiritual vessel.

When we regularly practice meditation and become proficient at quieting the mind, spiritual impulses permeate our mind and heart. Our understanding of life gradually takes on more and more of a spiritual perspective. We will find ourselves naturally attracted to other spiritual practices that deepen spiritual integration and relaxation.

Some forms of meditation have an element of contemplation. This occurs when we use a specific phrase or a mantra to focus our mind. The object of meditation is at once a focal point for stilling the mind and a spiritual seed that grows and flowers with each repetition.

In Christianity the Jesus prayer is used for meditation. The prayer "Lord Jesus Christ, have mercy on my soul" is repeated silently and coordinated with the breath. The mind focuses and quiets as concentration deepens. With each repetition, our consciousness is molded to appreciate the spiritual request expressed in the prayer. A vision of the sacred grows within us even as we calm and quiet the mind.

In the tradition of yoga there is a science of mantras. Certain mantras are believed to be appropriate for certain temperaments and personalities and to produce specific effects, while others are more general and can be used beneficially by anyone. An example of a general mantra is *so hum,* where the sound *so* is heard on the inhalation and the sound *hum* on the exhalation. This mantra translates as "that I am."

PATHWAYS TO THE SACRED

There are many more pathways to the sacred. Compassionate service can be a spiritual practice. Helping the poor, working for social justice, teaching, and healing are all forms of compassionate service. A pilgrimage to a holy and inspiring site is a way to experience the mystery of the sacred. Art, music, and writing can all be forms of spiritual expression and exploration.

This chapter is not meant to provide a complete list of all the pathways, but to give the reader samples of the most traveled spiritual paths. The challenge is to bring spiritual awareness into our daily life. When we do this, we develop a deep sense of peace, a strong feeling of connection, and vision and purpose in our life.

Art, music, and writing can all be forms of spiritual expression and exploration.

chapter twelve

---

relaxation

in

daily life

Y ou have explored five levels of relaxation. You have
learned a variety of relaxation techniques. Now
you are ready to begin the process of integrating these
techniques into your daily life. It is not enough to know
about relaxation, you need to practice it every day.

But you may have to overcome resistance before you
reach the goal of daily relaxation practice. It may feel overwhelming to add another activity to your busy schedule.

**You can reward
yourself for relaxation
practice by scheduling
an enjoyable activity
afterward.**

DAILY PRACTICE

One problem with starting a daily relaxation practice is that
we often have to give up something that seems pleasant
and undertake something that seems difficult. For example,
it may seem pleasant to sit on the couch, watch TV, and
munch chips. It may seem difficult to get up, exercise,
meditate, or practice diaphragmatic breathing.

There are several ways to overcome this inertia. Think
about relaxation practice in a way that makes it seem less
daunting. Ease into the practice by telling yourself that to
start you just need to do relaxation for five or ten minutes.
Tell yourself that you are just going to try it for a week or two.

You can reward yourself for relaxation practice by
scheduling an enjoyable activity afterward. Such an
incentive will help you to overcome your inertia.

You can practice relaxation in a pleasant setting, with

soothing music in the background and fresh air coming in the window. Vary your practice from day to day or week to week to keep it interesting. Keep a playful and creative approach.

It also helps when you become aware of the pleasant feelings accompanying relaxation. You can notice that it feels good to release muscular tension, to calm the autonomic nervous system, to let go of negative emotions, to center your mind. The experience of relaxation is inherently pleasant, while tension is ultimately painful. If you give yourself time to realize this, you will look forward to each relaxation session.

If you are able to practice relaxation every day for twenty-one days, you will have created a healthy habit. By then, relaxation practice will seem as natural as brushing your teeth or washing your face.

You can practice relaxation in a pleasant setting, with soothing music in the background and fresh air coming in the window.

INDIVIDUALIZING RELAXATION

There is no standard relaxation program that fits everybody. But there is a program of relaxation that is just right for you. You should pick a program that fits your situation, needs, and temperament.

Your choices about which relaxation method to use should be guided by the pattern of tension that you identified on the symptoms checklist in Chapter 1. For example, if you suffer from frequent tension headaches, muscular relaxation would be appropriate. If you have anxiety attacks, then breathing exercises, ANS, emotional, and mental relaxation techniques will be important. If emotional symptoms dominate, then you should use the techniques for emotional relaxation. If your mind is racing and chaotic, mental relaxation techniques are called for. If you feel isolated and empty, you might start with spiritual relaxation.

You have to consider your life situation when designing a relaxation program. If you have work and family commitments, you may need to select shorter practices that fit into your schedule. If you are older, walking or swimming might be good choices for exercise. If you are younger, vigorous exercise might fit into your relaxation program. If you are more introverted, then you may like to practice in solitude. If you are an extrovert, then you might enjoy a relaxation class.

Your daily relaxation program should include some form of direct relaxation practice such as those described in Chapters 3 and 5. Different elements can be blended into a single session of relaxation. You could start with diaphragmatic breathing, follow with differential relaxation, and conclude with concentration on the breath. Meditation blends muscular relaxation, breathing, mental focusing, emotional balancing, and spiritual harmony.

Exercise is a relaxation method that helps everyone.

If you have work and family commitments, you may need to select shorter practices that fit into your schedule.

Some active exercise
every day or even
every other day is a
very helpful part of
a complete relaxation
program.

Exercise reduces tension on many levels. Some active exercise every day or even every other day is a very helpful part of a complete relaxation program.

Component	Time	Options
Direct relaxation	1-2 times per day for 10-20 minutes	tense-release, differential, diaphragmatic breathing, autogenic training, 61 points, etc.
Exercise	20-30 minutes 3-4 times per week	Active: walking, biking, jogging, aerobics Passive: yoga stretches
Relaxation in action	2-3 minutes 3-5 times a day	3 diaphragmatic breaths, tension check and release, mindfulness, meditation in action
Spiritual relaxation	5-15 minutes daily 90 minutes once a week	prayer, read scriptures, compassionate service, meditation, worship

Daily stretching exercises can involve a few minutes in the morning and afternoon of desk exercises such as neck rolls, shoulder lifts, and overhead stretches. You can set aside thirty to sixty minutes several times a week to perform a thorough routine of stretching exercises.

A third component is relaxation in action. During the day's activities, you can learn to notice tension and to consciously relax. One way to practice relaxation in action is to anchor it to some specific event. After you conclude a phone call, take three even diaphragmatic breaths. Whenever you pass a certain landmark on your daily commute, check your breathing and let go of tension in your shoulders, neck, and face. Meditation in action can help you to maintain relaxation throughout the day.

Spiritual relaxation should also be a component of your daily relaxation practice. If you consider that the spiritual level is at the top of the relaxation hierarchy, and that spiritual relaxation eases tension on all the other levels, then you can see how important it is to have spiritual practice as part of your daily relaxation program.

Set aside a few minutes each day for prayer and the study of sacred scripture. You can have a daily period of meditation. You can dedicate time every day or week to formal worship. You can devote time each day to compassionate service. Daily spiritual practice will strengthen your belief and faith, deepen your sense of identity and purpose, and give you hope and optimism.

These four components of relaxation practice—direct relaxation techniques, exercise, relaxation in action, and spiritual practice—are the key building blocks for a complete relaxation program. You can use other techniques as need and situation arise. And you can vary the content of your daily relaxation practice to keep it fresh, interesting, and enjoyable.

A GOOD NIGHT'S SLEEP

Sleep is natural relaxation. It is the time when you cast off

> Direct relaxation techniques, exercise, relaxation in action, and spiritual practice are the key building blocks for a complete relaxation program.

the cares of daily living and completely relax both body and mind. During sleep, healing and restoration occur on all levels. After a good night's sleep, you feel refreshed and renewed.

At least, this is the way it should be. Unfortunately, sleep is often less than refreshing. The problem starts when you can't fall asleep at night. If you fall asleep, you can't stay asleep. You are tense and restless through the night. You wake up early or you struggle to get up in the morning. You feel tired throughout the day. You need a cup of coffee to get you started and sleeping pills to stop. Ultimately, you are denied the deep, natural relaxation sleep affords.

Fortunately, many behavioral strategies and relaxation techniques can help you fall asleep naturally and sleep peacefully through the night.

One obstacle to sleep is the use of caffeine. Caffeine is an effective stimulant that interferes with the natural pattern of sleep and wakefulness. You should try to avoid coffee and tea after midafternoon and drink no more than

During sleep, healing and restoration occur on all levels.

BEHAVIOR CHANGE	RELAXATION TECHNIQUES
Decrease caffeine	Direct Relaxation practice before bed
Eliminate nicotene	Guided relaxation in bed
Get up early	Even, smooth diaphragmatic breathing
Avoid daytime naps	2:1 breathing
Exercise daily	Use self-talks to reduce worries
Develop bedtime routine	Pleasant focus for mind

two cups a day. Anyone who has a real sleep problem should just eliminate caffeine. Nicotine is another strong stimulant that should be eliminated.

Daytime naps should be eliminated. Avoid late meals. Sleeping pills disrupt the quality of sleep and over time make sleep difficulties worse.

When you consider that you spend anywhere from a quarter to a third of your life sleeping, it makes sense to invest in a solid bed and a comfortable mattress. A warm but light covering can help to make sleep a comfortable experience. And you will probably rest best in natural fiber, i.e., cotton or silk sleepwear.

It also makes sense to invest the time, energy, and money to make your bedroom a pleasant and restful environment. Soothing colors and a clean, attractive room will make your bedroom a pleasant place to sleep.

Active exercise during the day helps to release tension and helps you to feel naturally tired. Relaxation practice can further reduce tension. Before you go to bed, take ten to twenty minutes to practice one of the direct relaxation techniques.

Once you get into bed, do a brief guided relaxation to let go of any lingering muscular tension. Then establish even, smooth diaphragmatic breathing. Move to 2:1 breathing, where the exhalation is twice as long as the

Soothing colors and a clean, attractive room will make your bedroom a pleasant place to sleep.

You need to use
your self-talks to
tell yourself that
late at night is not
a good time to
think about
your problems.

inhalation. A ratio of three or four counts with the inhalation and six or eight with exhalation works well for most people. The technique brings the body, nervous system, and mind to a quiet and peaceful state. Most people fall asleep after several minutes of 2:1 breathing.

The 2:1 breathing is the basis for a specific sleep exercise. Start by taking eight 2:1 breaths while lying on your back. Then, lying on the right side, taken sixteen 2:1 breaths. Finally, lying on the left side, take thirty-two 2:1 breaths. Most people fall asleep during this exercise. If you don't, then just repeat the procedure. If you still haven't fallen asleep, then continue with the 2:1 breathing.

Sometimes a tense and overactive mind can keep you awake. If so, you need to use your self-talks to tell yourself that late at night is not a good time to think about your problems. Every problem looks bigger and more ominous at night. Let go, and tell yourself that you will see how it looks in the morning. Or get up and write down your concerns. You may be surprised to find that worries which seemed to be huge, insurmountable problems during the dark of night actually seem pretty manageable in the light of day.

If your mind is consumed with negative thoughts about someone, use the technique of dwelling on the opposite. If you feel resentment toward someone, send feelings of compassion and understanding; if you feel anger, send feelings of love. This will help you release the negative thoughts and emotions keeping you awake.

Sometimes gently concentrating the mind helps. You can use the favorite place technique described in Chapter 5. Or go back through the events of the day, seeing them as you might on a videotape recorder, watching the events from early morning to evening. Recalling the progression of events concentrates your mind and helps you drift off to sleep.

A regular schedule can improve your sleep. Get up early in the morning, stay busy and active throughout the day, and go to bed at a reasonable time. Your schedule should allow you to get six to eight hours of sleep. Keep this schedule during the entire week. Don't sleep late on the weekend, because this makes it harder to fall asleep at a regular time on Sunday night.

Develop a bedtime routine. This routine might start by turning out the lights, checking the heat, taking the dog out, and turning on the dishwasher. Then do a few stretches and a relaxation, wash your face, brush your teeth, put on your pajamas, and go to bed. This routine will become a series of steps that naturally leads you to sleep.

Make sure you use your bed only for sleeping and making love. Don't work, read, talk on the phone, or watch TV in bed. You want to develop a conditioned link to your bed as a place to sleep, without associations with other activities.

If you find you can't fall asleep after utilizing relaxation and breathing exercises, get up, go to another room, and

Don't sleep late on the weekend, because this makes it harder to fall asleep at a regular time on Sunday night.